zodiaction

zodiaction

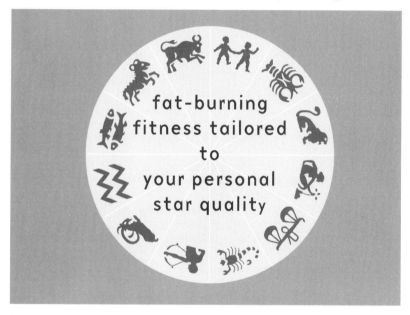

fat-burning
fitness tailored
to
your personal
star quality

by ELLEN BARRETT and BARRIE DOLNICK

BANTAM BOOKS

ZODIACTION
A Bantam Book / May 2007

Published by
Bantam Dell
A Division of Random House, Inc.
New York, New York

Zodiaction™ is a trademark of Barrie Dolnick and Ellen Barrett

Book design by Liney Li / 2eggsonaroll.com

Library of Congress Cataloging-in-Publication Data
Barrett, Ellen.
Zodiaction : fat-burning fitness based on your personal star quality /
Ellen Barrett and Barrie Dolnick.
p. cm.
ISBN 978-0-553-38437-6 (trade pbk.)
1. Physical fitness.   2. Astrology.   I. Dolnick, Barrie   II. Title.
RA781.B255 2007
613.7'10241335—dc22   2006037254

Printed in the United States of America
Published simultaneously in Canada

www.bantamdell.com

RRH   10 9 8 7 6 5 4 3 2 1

For those who look

at starry skies

and know that

all is possible

acknowledgments

I'm most grateful to my mother, Kitty, who introduced me to astrology way back when I was nine. You told me with enthusiasm that I was a Gemini, "a GREAT sign," and that Geminis were "smart and lucky." What a nice thing to say to an impressionable little girl.

Thanks to my sister and unofficial publicist, Sally, for rearranging the store shelves by placing my DVDs front and center. Now, that's love! I have no doubt you will be performing the same acts of "vandalism" with *Zodiaction*.

To my brother John, I owe my love of reading to you. You were always such a good influence. Thank you.

To my father, Kenny, for being a perfect example of Taurus—steady, down-to-earth and always home—thanks.

Thanks to my husband, Steve, the coolest guy in the universe. How did I land you? (My mom was right—*I really am smart and lucky!*)

To Barrie Dolnick, Jeremy Katz, and Philip Rappaport—the three best people to have around when you are attempting to write, sell, and edit a great book, thank you, thank you, and thank you.

To Beth Bischoff, our full-of-life photographer, and Glen Edelstein, our Art Director extraordinaire, thank you both so much.

And lastly, much gratitude goes to the women at my New Haven fitness studio for allowing me to incessantly interrogate and analyze you while writing *Zodiaction*. I know I asked "What's your sign?" one too many times. —**Ellen Barrett**

I would like to thank my co-author Ellen Barrett for her camera-ready expertise and irresistible workouts. Thank goodness for friends with humor—Cheryl Callan, Christine Chiocchio, Sheila Davidson, and Betsy Schecter, and thanks to my husband, Gero, and daughter Elisabeth for their good sense not to interfere. And last I offer gratitude to super-smart Jeremy Katz for his insight, and to Philip Rappaport and Glen Edelstein for shepherding this project with wisdom and charm.—**Barrie Dolnick**

contents

zodiaction

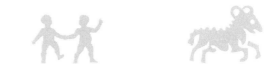

  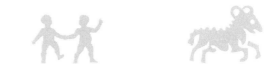

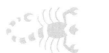

introduction

Have you ever wondered why you:

a. bought a membership to a yoga studio you never use?

b. hopped on the trend wagon and tried a Spin class you detested?

c. bought a ThighMaster, Abdominizer, or Slide 'n' Glide that now collects dust in your basement?

d. tried running every morning and ended up buying a donut instead?

Chances are you've answered "yes" to one or more of the above. That's because you were trying to fit into fitness.

Keeping fit and being healthy is not a function of keeping up with fitness trends or making yourself do exercises that you loathe. Being fit *now* is much more than a one-size-fits-all calorie-burning workout *and* a daily multivitamin because it's not just about the body. In this new age, we recognize that you have to add your mind and spirit into the wellness puzzle . . . and their interdependence is of crucial importance.

Once you know more about your natural talents, gifts, and foibles, you'll never waste your time on someone else's goals again.

Zodiaction offers an entirely new approach to fitness in which you start by knowing yourself and defining who you are—not just in body type or weight. We want you to know your strengths and use them to feel great. We want you to know your weaknesses and understand what triggers negative behavior.

Astrology offers you a unique basis for diagnosing your likes and dislikes, and your ability to stick to a routine, a diet, and a fitness plan. If you ever wondered why you prefer swimming to running, or why you need a game or competition to get you up and out, you're going to find out now. You will see that it's not only about what's best for workouts, but also your diet tendencies, your ability to work out with a buddy or a trainer, and your capacity to use your specialized astro-energy in the world at large.

Zodiaction offers customized fitness solutions based on the astrological signs (Aries, Taurus, Gemini, Cancer, Leo, Virgo, Libra, Scorpio, Sagittarius, Capricorn, Aquarius, Pisces). We assert that every person's perfect get-fit plan is already written in the stars. Each sign has its own particular quirks, strengths, and pitfalls, especially when it comes to being fit, healthy, and truly alive.

The sign of Taurus (April 20–May 20) for example, represents an earthy, fixed, luxury-loving, home-oriented person. The purchase of home workout equipment actually is a smart move for a Taurus. The more activities The Bull can do at home, the happier she is—that treadmill will definitely see some mileage. In contrast, if a Gemini (May 21–June 20) bought that equipment it would only be used as a clothing rack. Gemini thrives on getting out there, exploring, and seeking variety. If she had a home treadmill, she'd need a dozen books, a TV, and an iPod to keep her on it. For the most part a Gemini requires workout excitement.

Appreciating the differences among zodiac signs underscores why one exercise "routine" isn't good for everyone. Take Leo (July 23–August 22) vs. Pisces (February 19–March 20). Leo, The Lion, is king of the jungle, but in our instance, Leo is queen of the gym! Getting Lions to the gym requires no coercion, since they are known for their physical prowess. The Leo strength is their *strength*. They can handle tough workouts; they enjoy tough workouts; they want tough workouts—power yoga? high speed intervals around the track?—bring it on. Pisces, The Fish, doesn't have such sure footing in the gym. A major no-no when trying to motivate Pisces is use of the word "tough" to describe an upcoming workout. Pisces will go hide under a rock, never to be seen again. Pisces might prefer swimming, fluid yoga moves, or self-defense classes. Pisces people might burn calories worrying—so it's great to divert that expenditure of energy into more positive places.

Combining astrological characteristics with a fitness and diet strategy is natural synergy. Body parts have specific planetary rulers. Knowing how astrology and fitness work together opens a new door to overall self-awareness and wellness. *Zodiaction* is an irresistible combination of tools that has implications to every aspect of life—health, clarity, love, passion, creativity—it's all there. *Zodiaction* brings a novel integration of disciplines and evolves a deeper understanding of mind–body–spirit connection.

A Little Background

We work from two areas of expertise to bring you one smart fitness strategy. We combine over twenty years of experience interpreting the stars with fifteen years of cutting-edge fitness training and education.

ASTROLOGY

From an astrological standpoint, your sun sign stands for your karmic path—and influences everything in your life. If you're an Aries, you are in this world with Aries motives (be challenged, conquer, celebrate, repeat) and if you're here as a Cancer, you're entirely different (nurture, create safe havens, connect, love). Reading your daily horoscope is fine but that will not give you much insight about your true self. You probably know basic characteristics like "Leo loves to be in the limelight," but you might not know that "Leos hate to be cold so forget swimming in an unheated pool." You might be interested in learning why you just don't catch on to fitness fads "like everyone else does" or why your best friend is so attached to her couch. You will probably laugh at how accurately the signs describe your own behavior right off the bat. And once you trust that we know what we're doing, you'll find that our fitness suggestions are easy to take.

You may well wonder if twelve zodiac signs can be that different. The answer is a resounding *yes!* While writing this book we were impressed once again by how distinct each sign is when it comes to motivations, preferences, and attitudes.

To get you started with a little astrological background, here is a summary of the signs and what makes them tick. First, take a look at the chart below and then look up the corresponding element and modality for each sign.

SIGN	ELEMENT	MODALITY
Aries	Fire	Cardinal
Taurus	Earth	Fixed
Gemini	Air	Mutable
Cancer	Water	Cardinal
Leo	Fire	Fixed
Virgo	Earth	Mutable
Libra	Air	Cardinal
Scorpio	Water	Fixed
Sagittarius	Fire	Mutable
Capricorn	Earth	Cardinal
Aquarius	Air	Fixed
Pisces	Water	Mutable

Elements

Astrological signs fall under one of the four elements that, together, are necessary for life as we know it—fire, earth, air, and water. The elements stand for very separate and distinct qualities, and three signs fall under each element. Your sign's element gives you your first clue to a good mind-body-spirit connection. As you read about your sign, you'll see how this element is a building block toward the whole picture. Of course, it's just the beginning. Do you feel somehow connected to your element?

Fire is passion, creativity, and force—Aries, Leo, and Sagittarius are fire signs.

Earth is physical reality, abundance, and health—Taurus, Virgo, and Capricorn are earth signs.

Air is mind, communication, and concepts—Gemini, Libra, and Aquarius are air signs.

Water is emotional and intuitive—Cancer, Scorpio, and Pisces are water signs.

Modality

Each sign is also associated with a modality that describes its energy—how does your sign relate to action? Is your sign scattered or impatient, tolerant or stubborn? There are three modalities—cardinal (directed from one point to another), fixed (unmoving), and mutable (going in many directions). If you're a cardinal sign you like to go after goals on your self-approved strategy. Most of the time your drive takes you where you want to be but if your plan doesn't work, you typically have to start over because you're not interested in Plan B. If you're a fixed sign you take your own sweet time to do anything and it has to be on your terms. You might be called stubborn or inert when you don't make a move, but you're also patient when you need to be. A mutable sign is very flexible, which is great—but it's also very scattered and may not stick to a plan long enough to see it through.

When elements, modalities, and the basic characteristics of your sign are explored, you'll realize how important this information is in determining what your best mind–body–spirit balance is all about.

Here are some little teaser-tips for your best fitness strategy:

Aries—You like a challenge.

Taurus—You need to be in nice surroundings.

Gemini—As long as you're interested, you're happy.

Cancer—You need to trust your environment and the people in it.

Leo—It has to be fun!

Virgo—You need real information and benefits.

Libra—There can be no discord or ugliness.

Scorpio—You need something intense to hang on to.

Sagittarius—Action! Intrigue! Adventure!

Capricorn—You want a real goal and trackable results.

Aquarius—You need freedom, and the less crowded, the better.

Pisces—It has to be agreeable and without harsh lighting or tough talk.

After you read about your astrological profiles and get a good handle on the direction and strategies that work best for you, you'll be ready to embrace a smart, thorough workout program that will keep your body as fit as your mind and spirit.

zodiaction

Fitness

There are so many facets to fitness and well-being that we will wow you. This is not what you'd expect—not run-of-the-mill cardio, stretch, and strength. That's like describing a meal as food, liquid, and spice. There are infinite ways to make food, provide drink, and make it interesting, and the same goes for your workout. We have designed a five-star workout just for you and we know why you'll do it—because we totally understand you.

Zodiaction comes up with the fitness plan that works for your sign. We draw from yoga, treadmills, tennis courts, and mat classes. We intermingle disciplines that you may not have even heard of. We take that mind–body connection a step further by providing diet tips and spa therapy suggestions. Probably the most important thing we do is remind you that we totally understand what life's all about. You don't have to be pitch-perfect with *Zodiaction;* you only have to be true to yourself.

One fact holds true no matter what your sign: a balanced workout is ideal. Your astrological fitness disposition will take over from there and determine the specifics, but balance must be achieved first and foremost. With the stars as our guide, this balance won't be so difficult to maintain.

The Balance Triad

All successful workouts have three key components: cardiovascular training, strength training, and flexibility training, what we call *The Balance Triad*. You can go for each of these components separately or in combination, and you can focus on one more than the others, but excluding any one of the three will seriously throw you off track.

FIRST, A CARDIOVASCULAR TRAINING BREAKDOWN

It's defined as a system of physical conditioning designed to enhance circulatory and respiratory efficiency. You'll be training your heart (a very important muscle) to beat faster, increase body temperature, and break a sweat—sweating is good; it releases impurities and keeps you warm even when it's cold outside. Some signs like cardio more than others, but it's necessary for everyone.

Capricorn is a cardio all-star—The Goat likes to get into a steady heart-pumping zone and keep going. Taurus tends to loathe it—"It's uncomfortable," she whines—but needs it more than most. Then there's Gemini . . . she overestimates her lung capacity and needs to pay attention to breathing.

In the twelve *Zodiaction* workouts, cardio components vary in duration from ten minutes (Aquarius) to two hours (Capricorn). They vary in intensity, from light (Pisces) to hard core (Scorpio). They also require a variety of formats, from yoga (Leo) to boot camp (Sagittarius) to jumping rope (Libra). People tend to narrowly define cardio as jogging and swimming but just about anything can become cardiovascular-oriented. With the proper level of intensity, even Pilates and stretching can get you to sweat.

THE SECOND COMPONENT OF THE BALANCE TRIAD IS STRENGTH TRAINING

The next component of *The Balance Triad* is strength training—any exercise in which muscles contract, squeezing inward, is considered strength training. Typical results are either increased muscle strength or improved muscle tone. But dumbbells are not necessary! Gravity and body weight can provide perfect resistance too. For instance, in the Aries workout we use light-to-medium weights for a total body tone. In the Scorpio workout we use heavy weights for serious intensity. In the Cancer workout we go sans weights and do all on-your-side toning exercises. The Gemini workout doesn't include weights either, and the strength training is disguised as a dreamy ballet series.

You will not have to worry about whether or not you'll be able to do strength training and you should not have to stress over getting it done. Taking into account your zodiac sign pretty much guarantees we've figured out something you'll *want* to do—not just *have* to do.

THIRD POINT OF THE BALANCE TRIAD: FLEXIBILITY TRAINING

Last (but not least) is flexibility training, otherwise known as stretching. This component is comprised of exercises that tend to increase or maintain muscle and joint range of motion. We think it's the most underrated component, for stretching can really help with tension and toxin release, injury prevention, and overall agility. It also improves posture.

Zodiaction runs the gamut with stretching—it's not an afterthought or a cooldown staple. In fact, stretching is the first step in the Cancer workout. Flexibility training is sometimes performed standing (like in the Taurus workout) and sometimes seated (as in the Pisces workout). It can be ultra-Western (as in Sagittarius's sports conditioning–type stretches), or very Far-Eastern (like Leo's Ashtanga Yoga series). No matter the differences, the stretching technique complements the strength training and cardiovascular training components of each workout, completing *The Balance Triad.*

In essence, *Zodiaction* is the quintessential fusion fitness book, for here we not only fuse astrology with fitness, but also the mind with the body, and Eastern concepts with Western techniques. You'll see in the pages of this book that we celebrate just about everything, from Tae-Bo to Kundalini Yoga to Jack LaLanne calisthenics. We believe all of these exercise formats are ideal, for some sign, at some point. In this way, *Zodiaction* is inclusive and very modern. Just think, in the dawning of fitness training, a "one-size-fits-all" approach was standard. We've arrived at an exciting place, where now, customized workouts are the latest and greatest. *Zodiaction* is our way of providing you with your individualized workout prescription.

Signs of Other Life

While your first stop in *Zodiaction* will surely be your own sign, you are going to love reading all the signs that color your life.

YOUR OTHER SIGNS

Zodiaction is structured to guide you through your primary sign and then the other signs that influence your life. In astrology, there are separate signs that "rule" your love life, career, flirtation, and health. You'll be able to use the information within these signs to understand people around you and, to some extent, how you work in different situations. For example, if you feel stuck in your career and you see that it's ruled by the sign of Sagittarius, you could try a Sagittarian workout and see if that helps shift your energy to get unstuck. Same goes for health, love life, and flirtation. Don't be afraid to try the workouts under another sign if you think they might help you. The only rule we have in *Zodiaction* is to do something—anything—to keep active and aligned.

THE SIGNS OF OTHERS

Zodiaction also provides you with a glimpse into why your best friend always wants to take tango classes (Leo) or won't get off that couch (Taurus). We all like a little insight into the people we love and we know that you'll get a peek at the people in your life when you read their signs. Even better, if you understand why your sister is so unwilling to go running with you, you will stop being disappointed. You might even find a common interest or sport you can do together that will appeal to you both. *Zodiaction* promotes peaceful and harmonious relationships through healthy understanding of individual motivations.

Be Smart

We're not trying to replace your doctor or your trainer. They've worked with you firsthand and know you well, so we beg you—don't dump them for us! Take *Zodiaction* for what it is—a fun, inspiring kick in the pants that may assist you in achieving weight loss, total fitness, and workout harmony once and for all.

You have all you need to make *Zodiaction* work for you. Have fun staying fit!

aries-action

THE RAM March 21–April 19

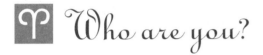 Who are you?

In One Word: AMBITIOUS

Symbol(s): A geyser; ram's horns. The Aries energy is bursting forth, pushing through.

Color: Fire-engine red!

Element: FIRE. This is a purifying element that typically gives out heat. Fire can be destructive when it runs rampant and destroys whatever is in its path. But fire is also very useful when it provides the energy for productivity. Fire signs are active and they like a good fight/challenge/competition. It's important to win. Aries hates to lose and it can really show.

Energy: CARDINAL. This means that its energy flows out like an arrow toward a target. Once you have a goal in mind, a strategy is developed and a plan is executed—just hope that no one is in the way. Your cardinal energy can steamroll an elephant and you won't even notice. Your cardinal energy brings the need for goal-oriented workouts so you have something to work toward.

Psychic Domain: Aries rules the ego. It is a very independent sign—but with typical paradox, the spiritual task of Aries is to remember that the other person may not pack the same degree of heat. In other words, Aries must learn to get along with others rather than feel challenged by them.

Physical Domain: Aries rules the head. You can bet you'll get headaches with stress. You probably don't mind the head hit in soccer and volleyball and if you lose a few teeth in hockey, oh well. You're a good sport about your own injuries but don't always apologize when you cause them in others.

What to Avoid in the Aries Workout: Wussy workouts, people who talk about their injuries, slowpokes, bossy teammates.

Ideal Workout: Three qualities are essential for Aries. First, you like to track progress. It's not just about achieving something measurable; Aries cares about the process of how she got from A to Z. Second, you enjoy cardiovascular activity. Third, The Ram likes to roam. Don't pen yourself in. Workouts such as cycling, hiking, and running are great.

Essential Workout Gear: Cross-training sneakers and a riding helmet.

Ultimate Trouble Spot: Arms—keeping them from injury!

Workout Buddy Warning: Don't be late and keep up the pace. Constant talking isn't necessary. Expect long periods of silence—that's just The Ram's independent nature.

If You Have a Personal Trainer:

1. Make sure he/she knows you like to be challenged!

2. Ask for a workout strategy for at least an eight-week period; you need goals.

3. Suggest as much outdoor training as possible; you'll work harder.

Strategic Choices for Aries

The Aries Diet: As an Aries, you eat to have energy to achieve your goal. *Fuel* is The Ram's dietary buzzword. Beware of protein-heavy diets like Atkins. Protein is slow to digest, taking considerable time to convert into accessible energy. You (and your body) are impatient and need a quicker turnaround. So be sure to have some carbohydrates at every meal. You'll thrive on fruits and whole grains. Breakfast is your crucial meal—make it oatmeal and O.J. or whole grain toast and organic jam. There is no doubt healthy carbs should start your day.

Aries does not have a delicate digestive system. You can eat just about anything.

You'll try what pleases you and you don't use the word "diet" a whole lot. Yes, you do have a sweet tooth. The single serving or "bite-size" samplers are a good choice for you. You should definitely treat yourself to these treats (they tend to be instant energy), but in the right amount, which is *moderate*. Buying and then eating sweets in bulk will cause you to short circuit. Your sugar high will plummet to a sugar low, taking Aries out of the running. Yikes!

Are you an Aries who wants to lose weight? If so, no need to consult a dietician, join Weight Watchers, or recruit a weight-loss buddy. Like with everything else, The Ram is very independent. It's best to travel the weight-loss road on your own. When you set your mind to it, you lose weight. It's that simple. You don't need the outside "support" like many of the other astrological signs do.

Tempting as it is, food on the go is not what's best for Aries. When life gets very busy, your eating habits and weight can go two different ways—up or down. Unlike Libra, Aries tends to put on weight with a busy schedule. A tight schedule isn't all that stressful for you; it's the norm.

Your food choices become less than stellar, though. Planning ahead might be tough, but taking a stash of homemade snacks on the road every day is better than that gas-station burrito. Junk food is okay now and then—you'll burn it off. But any Aries who indulges in too many preservatives and prepackaged meals will lose her coveted edge.

THE TOP THREE ITEMS TO SHOP FOR:

1. **Hot and cold cereal.** Like Seinfeld, you love it for snacking, for lunch, and you sometimes eat it dry.

2. **Staple fruits.** Apples, bananas, oranges, grapes . . . you like the tried-and-trues. Aries can't go for long periods of time without eating, and fruit is a great on-the-go energy boost.

3. **Ice cream, Creamsicles, Popsicles,** *gelati.* You're hot fire-engine red, remember? You do a lot of heart-pumping and blood-boiling things. You love cold foods because they cool you down.

Diet Vice: Tequila shots.
Signature Spa Treatment: Scalp massage.

zodiaction

Complementary Therapy: Sacral-cranial balancing.
Mindfulness Mantra: Vulnerability is not weakness.

Aries has the whole take-no-prisoners fearless warrior thing down. What's missing is comfort with normal human vulnerability. A mindful Aries recognizes feelings of compassion, fear, sensitivity, and fragility in herself and others. Everyone is vulnerable in some way, every day. Aries women typically forge through uncomfortable feelings by focusing on things they can accomplish.

Learn to be at ease with your entire emotional range. Embrace your inner coward, let yourself feel fear. It's okay to be insecure. When you let yourself soften, others will find you more approachable. Your friends know you've got a big heart and that you'd do anything for them. When you need them, you can let them be there for you too.

Aries in a Nutshell

MIND: Think first, act later? Nah. You are a doer. You'll take action—sometimes impulsive action—over long, weighty consideration. Try to listen to your inner thoughts and feelings now and then, especially when you want to move on something very quickly. You have so much spiritual intelligence, but you have to listen to it in order to use it.

BODY: Aries needs to shake off energy and "create" accomplishment by seeing hard numbers. Aries likes to know her body-fat composition. She wants to know how many miles she just ran on the treadmill. If she's taking a karate class, she wants to know how close she is to achieving that black belt.

SPIRIT: You are the world's spiritual warrior. Your energy and drive set a high standard for can-do/will-do women. You can accomplish anything you want—and you know it.

Be selective about your causes and compassionate in your battles.
Be wise when you accept your winnings and at ease when you need a helping hand.

An Aries Workout Story

Clare, a CEO of an import/export company, was born under the sign of Aries on April 5. She has climbed the corporate ladder and is a well-paid, powerful executive. On one particular sunny Saturday, Clare set out to climb a different ladder—the yogi ladder. Clare attended a Hatha Yoga class for the first time.

Yoga is all about breathing, stretching, and concentrating your focus on your breath: you stretch, you zone. Yoga is not a sport. But Clare was overcome by her Aries sense of competition. Her eye wandered around the class, scouting out her "opponents," checking out the fancy poses and buff bodies. Her frustration mounted as those around her blissfully exhaled back into Downward-Facing Dog. Clare kept glancing at the clock as if locked in a prison cell. "Let's pick up the pace," she mumbled to herself. Clare's stress levels increased, contrary to the intention of yoga.

After class, when everyone else was sauntering out in calm, centered clarity, Clare wanted to debrief. She talked about every other person in the class, whether they were better or worse than she. Her yoga experience was a comparison between herself and her fellow students, devoid of "tuning in." The powerful breathing, the soothing stretches, and the peaceful vibe of yoga were all lost on Ms. Competitive. The end result was a failing grade in yoga 101.

Sometimes the Aries competitive streak is a positive attribute for fitness, great for Spin class or playing in a tennis league. Competition can push you into a more advanced level. In the yoga studio, however, it's a bit of a blemish, where the Aries competitive nature can backfire, losing all workout benefit. If you see your Aries-self in Clare, learn how to turn off your competitive switch when necessary.

THE ARIES "IN IT TO WIN IT" WORKOUT

All successful workouts have three key components: strength training, cardiovascular training, and flexibility conditioning. You can go for each of these separately or in combination, but excluding any one of the three is an absolute no-no in *Zodiaction*. Balance is always the way to go, no matter what sign you were born under.

As a Ram, it is very important for you to work out, not necessarily to lose weight, but to combat stress and to rid your body of excess energy. You know that temper of yours? Of course you do. Exercise is a much healthier release than popping someone in the nose or saying something you'll later regret. You are simply a better person to be around when you let off some steam by working out regularly. If you don't believe us, ask your friends.

Many of the other astrological signs require tons of goading when it comes to cardio, but not Aries. You are attracted to heavy breathing, like a moth to a flame, and you especially like to run or power walk outdoors. Stomping around is therapeutic. To roam free with the wind on your face, and "charge" forward with a sprint every now and then . . . this is something you'll do instinctively, even joyfully. Heart-pumping exercise makes you feel alive!

The Ram is strong, but lacks balance within that strength. A good example of this is the Aries spinner. (Spinning is something that Aries are drawn to, so this may specifically pertain to you.) By logging many hours in cycling class, your hamstrings have been overdeveloped, while your upper back muscles remain underdeveloped. A big goal for the Aries workout is to even out the muscles of the body. You don't need to "get stronger." You simply need to "get more symmetry." A truly healthy body possesses muscular harmony. You'll pay attention to every major muscle of the body.

Stretching tends to be Aries' Achilles' heel. You lack the patience to hold stretches long enough to really improve your flexibility. Aries perceives stretching as a waste of time, as though you could be doing something else more productive. Slow doesn't mean worthless, pal. Slow movement helps remove lactic acid (a natural by-product from muscle activity) and prevents injury. No need to hurt yourself by being in a hurry.

THE ARIES WORKOUT HAS THREE PARTS

1. "Freedom" Cardio

Have you ever seen a ram at the zoo? He looks miserable confined in that limited space. When the ram's freedom is compromised, his spirits sag. As a Ram yourself, you probably can relate to the emotional discomfort of cramped quarters, which is why you thrive on freedom—cardio! This means cardiovascular exercise that travels, with little or no confinement to equipment or space. Outdoor running, biking, kayaking, hiking, or Rollerblading are some good examples of "freedom cardio" that are perfect for this high-energy, independent sign. If you live in a wintry environment, perhaps taking up cross-country skiing or snowshoeing will be to your liking.

2. Total Body Sculpt

We'll use light-to-medium sized handheld weights (3–8 lb each) and hit every major muscle of the body to subtle fatigue. Free-weights, as opposed to Nautilus machinery, are best—remember, nothing should confine The Ram. The number of repetitions will vary from person to person and muscle group to muscle group, depending on one's threshold for fatigue. This is one of the best ways to promote muscular symmetry.

3. Timed and Multitasking Stretch

Yes, a stopwatch will come in handy—we'll be holding stretches for no less than sixty seconds, which will undoubtedly be your biggest workout challenge. Luckily, we are going to stretch two or more muscle groups at once. This will appeal to The Ram's need for accomplishment. It'll also save time. A total of eight stretches, held for one minute each, is all that is needed. (Keep reminding your Aries-self that stretching matters!)

WORKOUT PRESCRIPTION

Aries is ambitious and overflows with energy at times. For these two reasons, the *Aries Workout Prescription* is five to six days per week. You'll have at least one full day off from any formal workout. Knowing Aries, your day(s) off will be anything but idle. Household chores, childcare, or hobbies will keep you moving a bit. Be sure to take a day! The typical Aries injury is a result of pushing too hard and resting too little. The variety in your routine really comes in the form of cardiovascular activity that you choose. Try to mix it up! Cycling too many days in a row tends to be too much of a good thing.

Aim for:

- cardiovascular training: five times per week
- strength training: three times per week
- flexibility training: three times per week

If you're an Aries exerciser in a gym, be sure to snag the treadmill that is near a window. Looking outside will help you stay motivated. You aren't that gung ho about group exercise classes, but a great way to get cardio on a rainy day is to enroll in a Salsa, Swing, or Step class. These could be great "backups" every now and again.

zodiaction

BEST TIME TO WORK OUT: After work when you want to hit someone.

STEP 1: Cardio (approximately 30–60 minutes). Get some cardiovascular activity, preferably outside. You are very independent, so lace up those sneakers and go solo.

STEP 2: Strength Training (approximately twenty minutes). Perform the total body strength training moves below, in the showcased sequence. Do however many repetitions are needed to fatigue the targeted muscle. You'll know you've hit your fatigue when your form becomes sloppy and the weight feels very, very heavy. When your muscles begin to shake, it's time to move on.

Shoulder Press

(TONES THE MUSCLES SURROUNDING THE SHOULDERS)

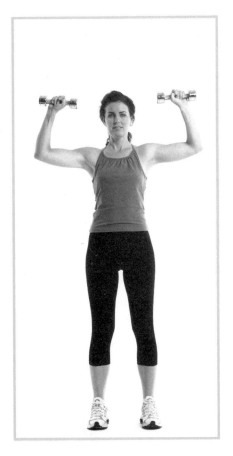
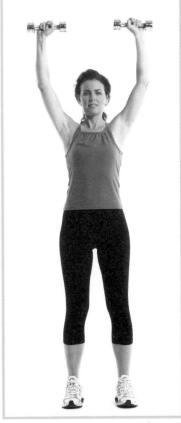

Stand with feet together and abdominals engaged. With one weight in each hand, bend elbows and bring hands up to shoulder level.

Exhale and simultaneously extend both arms straight up. Repeat at a moderate pace until shoulders feel fatigued.

Biceps Curl

(TONES THE UPPER ARM MUSCLES)

Stand with your feet together and engage your abdominals. Bring weights down and in front of you, palms facing up.

Exhale and bend the elbows, bringing the weights up toward each shoulder. Inhale and return to the starting position. Repeat at a moderate pace until the biceps fatigue.

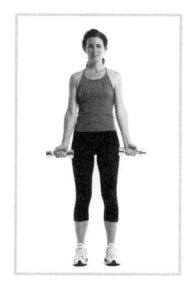
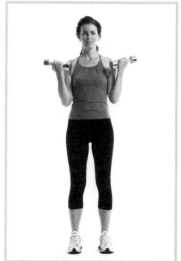

Standing Leg Scissor

(TONES THE INNER AND OUTER THIGH MUSCLES)

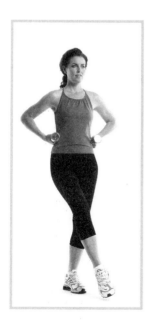
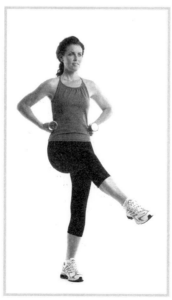

Bring the weights down to the waist and stand firmly on your left leg. Extend the right leg to the front along the floor.

Exhale and, as if you were kicking a soccer ball, lift the right leg up and "scissor" across the body. Keep hips square to the front. Repeat swiftly, until the right leg muscles fatigue. Then repeat the entire exercise on the other side.

Reverse Fly

(STRENGTHENS THE UPPER BACK MUSCLES)

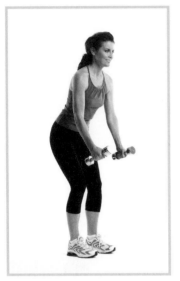 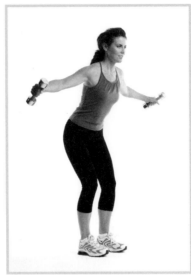

Stand with the feet together, knees slightly bent, lean forward, but keep back straight. Keep a micro-bend at the elbows and firm wrists.

Exhale and, lifting both arms up and back, squeeze the shoulder blades together. Repeat at a moderate pace, until the upper back fatigues.

Tiptoe Lunge

(AN EXCELLENT EXERCISE FOR STRONGER THIGH MUSCLES)

Start with your left leg forward and your right leg back. You'll be up on your toes on the right side, so balance is a challenge right from the start. Keep your torso upright, and allow your arms (with one handheld weight in each hand) to drop to the side.

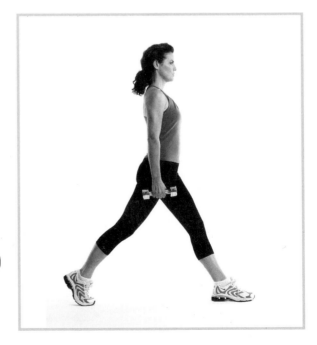

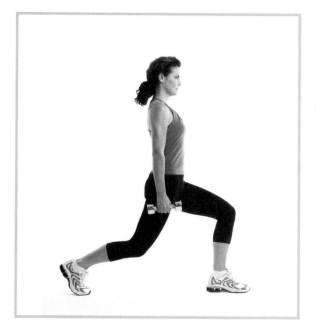

Inhale and bend both knees. Exhale and straighten back to the starting position. Repeat again and again at a moderate pace until the leg muscle shows signs of fatigue. Be sure to repeat the entire exercise with the right leg forward.

Double Crunch

(A VERY EFFECTIVE ABDOMINAL EXERCISE)

Lie on your back with both feet off the floor and both hands behind your head. Knees are stacked over the hips. Exhale and simultaneously lift the hips and the shoulders off the ground, crunching the abdominals. Inhale and return to the starting position. Repeat at a swift pace until the core muscles feel fatigued.

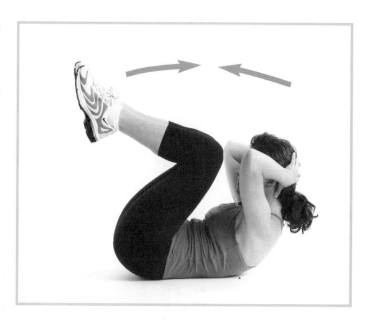

zodiaction

STEP 3: Stretching (approximately ten minutes). It's time to slowly stretch. Hopefully, the aforementioned exercise has snuffed out your Aries restlessness. Much like in Step Two, the stretch series for Aries is total body, hitting all of the major muscles.

Turtle Stretch

(STRETCHES AND DE-STRESSES THE MUSCLES SURROUNDING THE SPINE)

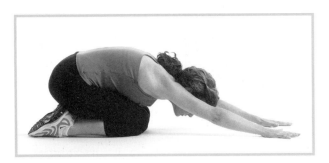

Kneel down, with knees and ankles together. Try to keep hip-to-heel contact and drape the upper body forward and down. Extend the arms up overhead. Feel a nice release of tension in the lower back and a subtle stretch in the front thigh.

Janu Sirsasana

(THIS IS A YOGA POSE THAT TRANSLATES AS "HEAD TO KNEE" AND IT'S A VERY EFFECTIVE WAY TO STRETCH THE HAMSTRINGS)

This is a great yoga pose that simultaneously stretches the hamstrings and back. Extend your left leg straight and bend your right knee. The sole of the right foot should lightly press on the left inner thigh. Turn your torso so it lines up with the

extended leg. Now take your hands and slowly "walk" them down the leg until you feel a challenging stretch. Eventually, your forehead will make contact with your knee. Hold for sixty seconds. Repeat with right leg extended.

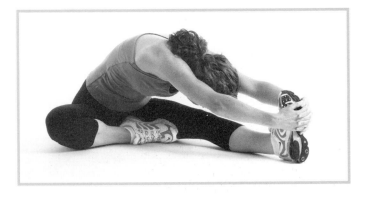

Straddle Stretch

(STRETCHES THE MUSCLES OF THE RIGHT AND LEFT THIGHS SIMULTANEOUSLY)

Sit on the floor and extend both legs out at a wide angle, creating a "V." The knees can be bent or straight, whatever feels better. Now take your hands in front, keep your back straight (no hunching), and lean forward. The stretch should be apparent right away. Breathe calmly and hold for one full minute. Use your hands for support.

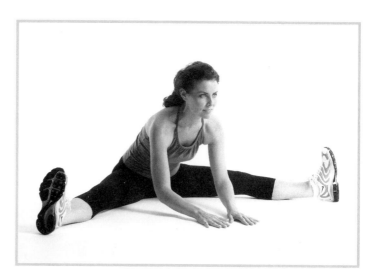

Spine Twist

(HELPS IMPROVE LOWER BACK FLEXIBILITY)

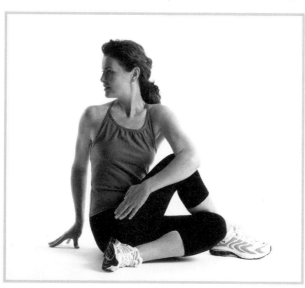

This is essential—in some form or another—for every astrological sign. Sit on the floor with your left leg bent underneath the right leg. Place the sole of the right foot on the floor behind the left knee. Now exhale and twist the torso to the right, ideally bringing the left forearm across to the outer right thigh. Hold for sixty seconds with calm, smooth breaths and then repeat on the other side.

Cobra Stretch

(IMPROVES LOWER, MIDDLE, AND UPPER BACK FLEXIBILITY AND STRETCHES THE ABDOMINALS)

Lie on your belly with the palms of your hands underneath the shoulders.
Inhale and press the body up, "peeling" the rib cage off the mat. Look up and
breathe. Hold for sixty seconds and then exhale and release.

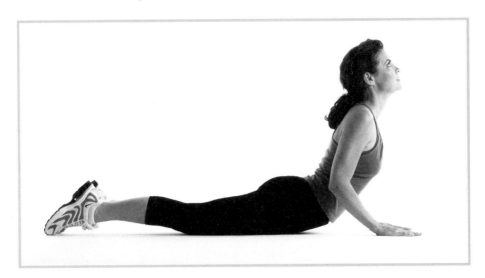

What's Ahead of Aries: A Star-Driven Five-Year Plan

2007   Lots of energy, exuberance, and curiosity. You're a spiritual warrior. Can you
learn how to have fun and not suffer from overdoing it? Can you compete
without injuring yourself or your pride? Focus on being your true self in the
fall.
Key Workout: Long walks in new neighborhoods.

2008   Seriously, you're onto a big idea this year. Your ambition is in full throttle
and working those long hours can be a challenge. Can you find a way to
balance hard work with working out? The stars say you might get
sidetracked. Don't neglect your health!
Key Workout: Machines that let you read or watch the news.

2009   Wacky-doodle-do! You're into new stuff this year, some a little off the beaten path. Whether it's parasailing or extreme desert hiking, you're all about pushing out of your comfort zone. Just don't abandon your friends too long; they'll want to try to keep up.
       Key Workout: Dance competitions.

2010   Welcome to Making Balance Work. This year is about you and someone close to you getting along, getting closer, getting to the heart of the matter. Don't give up on love. Put down your weapon and put on your diplomacy. Ultimately, you'll enjoy having a companion to walk (or run) with.
       Key Workout: Moving meditation.

2011   This is YOUR YEAR. Luck is with you. You're all energy and focus and drive. Nothing stops you. Expansion is your key word—but watch the waistline. Celebrating can have side effects.
       Key Workout: You choose. It's all good.

Signs of Life

Aries isn't your only sign by a long shot. In your solar chart, each sign rules a different part of your life. You can get to know the energetic qualities of your life if you take some time to explore signs outside of your own. You can even try the kind of workouts that appeal to them. You'll experience how walking a mile in someone else's shoes can bring you wisdom and appreciation for the differences among us.

Read about these signs if you want some insight into other parts of your life:

Love life—Libra

Career—Capricorn

Flirtation—Leo

Health—Virgo

taurus-action

THE BULL April 20–May 20

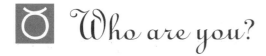 *Who are you?*

In One Word: STEADY

Symbol(s): A bull's horns. The Taurus energy is sturdy, persistent, practical, and composed. Sturdy as a bull, stubborn as a bull.

Color: Irish green

Element: EARTH. Physical life, abundant land, comfort and luxury—this is Taurus, the sign of earthly delights. This is the energy that makes things real—it's about construction, acquisition, and tangible assets. Physical health is a function of earth, but so is a good couch. Sometimes it's a battle between being in your element or receding into it. The struggle is basically lifelong. Who wins—you or the couch? It's up to you.

Energy: FIXED. Three guesses what that means. And if you answer stubborn, unmoving, or lazy, you're right. Being a fixed sign is awesome for sticking to your guns. But it's also the evil twin to go-for-it health and fitness. Taurus has to discipline The Bull so that he doesn't dig into a rut. Even immoveable earth needs to renew itself with some fresh air, water, and sunshine.

Psychic Domain: Taurus rules stuff—money, real estate, clothing, furniture,

Tupperware, anything you can get your hands on. Taurus is a sign engaged in practicality and the pursuit of comfort. Hey, that's a good thing. You love to look good and if that's enough motivation to stay fit, you're good to go. Beware of exercise that looks too easy: it is.

Physical Domain: Taurus rules the neck and throat. Make sure you are warm and keep yourself hydrated to avoid sore throats. Those scarves aren't just showing your stylish flair; when your neck is warm, the rest of your Taurus body is warm and toasty too. Tension and stress settle in the neck and jaw. It's important not to hold back on what you need to say. You have naturally good health and stamina but you have to use it. If cooking and eating were a sport you'd get Olympic gold.

What to Avoid in the Taurus Workout: Unpleasant surroundings (like smelly gyms), uber-competitors (like hardcore Spin classes), and take-no-prisoners instructors (just say no to anything "boot camp").

Ideal Workout: Taurus needs a workout that is thorough and gentle. Extra credit goes to workouts you can do at home—as long as you *do* them. Those in-home walking DVDs? Great option for Taurus! And any kind of in-your-body, get-the-job-done stretching and strengthening is nice too. Panting and sweating are optional. Big breathing, however, is mandatory. We want to see your lungs expand.

Essential Workout Gear: Totally cute athletic footwear. Dirty, old sneakers will snuff out your enthusiasm to exercise, while the hottest *must-haves* will do the opposite—you'll gladly work out with those happy feet! Is there a moral to this story? Taurus—don't feel guilty next time you splurge on the latest footwear or electronic gizmo.

Ultimate Trouble Spot: Thighs and butt area.

Workout Buddy Warning: Taurus is independent—you don't need a companion to work out with, but you do like the guilt-producing pangs of a partner who keeps you on your fitness program. A good friend who won't give in to your desire for pizza instead of Pilates is what you need but stay clear of anyone the least bit judgmental or a speedster. You'll have none of that.

If You Have a Personal Trainer:

1. Make sure your trainer knows you need to be gently coaxed. You are utterly turned off by any sort of whistle blowing, foul language, or unattractive terminology like "gastrocnemius." (Please, just say "calf muscle.")

2. Make sure you insist on a realistic goal right from the start—something easy to track, like a reasonable weight or possible size. Your trainer needs to remind you of your eye-on-the-prize goal every single time you meet.

3. Your trainer has to be cute.

Strategic Choices for Taurus

The Taurus Diet: As a Taurus, eating is pleasure, and the Food Network might be your porn. Forget fuel. You want to enjoy really good food in a nice atmosphere, but something fast and satisfying will do too. Taurus is the sign of the gourmand. You can't help it! You know what's good, better, and best. But it is very easy to indulge and that's where The Bull needs some training.

Taurus is naturally intuitive about health. You know what agrees with you and what is just not good, but sometimes immediate gratification wins over self-discipline. You can avoid that by having a variety of yummy snacks at your fingertips daily. That way, you won't be as tempted by a prepackaged cupcake when you're buying your Evian water.

THE TOP THREE ITEMS TO SHOP FOR:

1. **Fresh fruit, specifically oranges, apples, and melon.** These are fairly low-calorie, no-fat, water-based fruits that are great for cleaning the digestive tract. You're an earth sign, which demands careful and conscious tending. "Live" food heightens your energy and fills you up. Your skin will glow and your waist will shrink. You don't want a drought or rain forest; you want to be a healthy, beautiful garden.

2. **Salad greens (not the pale and nutrient-devoid iceberg lettuce), specifically the deeper green leaf lettuces, romaine, and arugula.** Salad greens are great roughage; they enable Taurus to eat the bigger quantity of food that satisfies you, without intaking excess calories. These veggies are good sources of beta-carotene too—and remember, the darker the color of the salad green, the more nutritious it is.

3. **Legumes, specifically chickpeas and black beans.** These are high-fiber complex carbohydrates. Hummus and bean dip straight up or added to salads are great nibbly items to satisfy The Bull's carb cravings with intelligence. They'll boost your energy, yet don't pollute your body with excess sugars.

The important thing for Taurus to remember about diet is this: you love not just to eat, but to *feast*. The only way you can eat large quantities of food and keep your weight down is to fill up on good stuff, like fruits and veggies and whole grains. (Thank God dessert is served last. You may be full by then, and have just a bit!) A very restricted diet is a total no-no. You'd rather jump off a cliff.

Diet Vice: The bread basket.
Signature Spa Treatment: Swedish massage.
Complementary Therapy: Nutrient-rich mud baths.
Mindfulness Mantra: I have all that I need.

Taurus is the "I Have" sign of the zodiac and dislikes even the concept of "Have Not." When a Taurus is feeling stressed, under attack, emotionally down, or some other blah, uncomfortable feeling, there are two easy but not-so-good fixes: eating and shopping. Eating is literally feeding yourself to compensate for what you think you don't have. Shopping is looking for external patches to internal holes. Taurus has amazing patience and fortitude, so if these sisters of virtue can be called upon to help out when you're down, you won't end up with too-tight jeans and debt-heavy credit cards. Your strength is in your very nature: I Have . . . all that I need. I Have beauty, power, patience, and the wisdom to know that discomfort transforms itself without chocolate or cashmere. Taurus knows all it needs to know, but it's just kind of nice to be reminded once in a while.

Taurus in a Nutshell

MIND: If it feels good, do it. The easy road does not require any effort. It's the stuff that doesn't feel so good that gets in the way. You bring the gift of manifestation and physical beauty into this world. It's wasteful if you don't put those gifts to use. It's hard to shake off inertia, so don't even get to that point. Keep your energy and purpose in motion and we'll all get to benefit by your good taste and exemplary behavior.

BODY: Taurus has a lovely body that likes to be stretched, massaged, pampered, and worshipped. One of the most grounded signs on the planet, Taurus is our earthly beauty, our Goddess bounty. Taurus is fertile, tactile, and delicious. Taking care of this body includes movement, fluidity, and energy—it's important that a Taurus balances pleasure with practicality.

SPIRIT: You are the world's connection to fruitful abundance. Your energy is steady, resilient, and powerful. We all want to be around a healthy Taurus because your aura is healing.

Share your life force with us by taking care of yourself and being out in the world.

Be happy with yourself and your possessions; enjoy the freedom in generosity.

A Taurus Workout Story

Mira is a sleep-till-noon type. She's also a Taurus. Coincidence? No. Basking in one's comfy bed is typical Bull. When Mira started to put on the "freshman fifteen" in college, her totally adorable, absolutely beloved Calvin Klein jeans stopped fitting her. That sent her on a workout search—she knew she had to do something. (A life without those jeans was a sad, sad notion.) So Mira signed up for a nine o'clock in the morning Tae-Bo class that met three times per week. She paid $250 for a semester's worth of Tae-Bo, then scurried to the Nike Outlet for some apparel. She was ready to kick and punch and Tae and Bo.

Mira attended one class. That's it. Just one class. February, March, April, and May came and went. She enjoyed the one class she went to, but the comfort of her 500-thread count sheets was too enticing. Mira never got her butt out of bed.

The first lesson to be learned here is this: *know thyself.* Eighteen-year-old Mira didn't quite know herself enough; she was still discovering who she is, what makes her tick. (Hopefully she learned a bit about her tendencies on her Tae-Bo adventure.) Taurus usually doesn't wake up with lightning bolts of energy.

The second lesson to be learned is this: the time of day you opt to work out is often just as important as the type of workout. Be sure it's a time of day when your energies are soaring.

zodiaction

THE TAURUS "CONSISTENCY WINS" WORKOUT

Taurus doesn't bore easily—a great attribute—if The Bull finds an exercise that she likes, she won't compulsively search for "the next best thing" (. . . unlike some other signs we know). That twenty-minute walking loop around your neighborhood will do just fine, over and over again. The secret is to ACTUALLY DO IT!! And at least three times a week. Taurus, we know your intentions are good: you "get" that you need to work out and you write it on your to-do list in pen. But more than any other sign, something happens between *thinking about* working out and *actually* working out. *Zodiaction*'s job is to nip that in-between area in the bud; nothing shall come between you and your workout! Your motivation is simple: you want to look good and be comfortable. Well, you won't look good or feel comfortable dragging around extra weight. So come on . . . let's get to our workout.

Remember, no matter what your sign, the workout must be balanced and that means there are three parts: strength, stretch, and cardio (not necessarily in that order). Taurus needs to emphasize cardio—simple, steady movement that gets your blood pumping and skin glistening. Thus, cardio is 75 percent of your ideal routine.

THREE WORKOUT GOALS FOR TAURUS

1. The workout needs to be simple—the "do-it-anywhere/rely-on-no-one" workout—because you need to actually JUST DO IT at least three times a week.

2. Find the right intensity that makes you purr. If the workout is too intense you'll dread it. And window shopping is not intense enough. Pay attention to the perfect level of intensity—something you can stick with.

3. Reward yourself with something new to wear once you hit that goal. Clothing and accessories are ultra-motivating to Taurus.

WORKOUT PRESCRIPTION

Taurus The Bull can take on a challenge, but that means getting up a head of steam and devising a strategy. The best way to avoid failure is to make a plan you can follow. Forget fads. Forget the Spin class special of ten classes for the cost of eight—it doesn't save you any money if you never go! Think of your fitness plan as a personal shopper that makes you move well instead of dress well. It's all about your body, the most amazing, miraculous thing you own. Reframe the idea of the workout—it's more of a "Body Polish."

Get into nature, connect to the earth, and bow to the universe. It comes naturally to you when you don't think of it like your high school gym class.

BEST TIME TO WORK OUT: In the late morning, or you won't do it at all.

STEP 1: Low-Key Fat-Burning Training (forty-five minutes in duration). Set a steady pace and go. Your indoor cardio can take the form of a treadmill, Elliptical, StairMaster, or stationary bike. It can also be outdoors: a hike, a bike ride, or a long walk. The key is to be steady and keep it low-impact, which means no running, no sprinting, and whatever you do stay away from crazy-steep inclines. The pace should be moderate. Don't stop for a swig of water either; drink as you move. Keep moving, Taurus . . . for forty-five solid minutes. *Bodies at rest stay at rest, bodies in motion stay in motion.* We want you to stay in motion for forty-five minutes!

STEP 2: Simple Strength. No equipment is needed for these five true-blue calisthenics. These should be performed immediately following your cardio jaunt.

Simple Squat

(STRENGTHENS THE BUTTOCK AND THIGH MUSCLES)

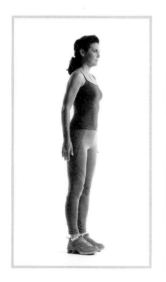
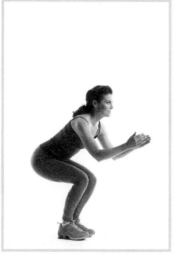

Stand tall with feet parallel, arms down by your sides.

Now bend both knees simultaneously, as if sitting in a chair. Return to starting position. Repeat ten times total at a moderate pace. Allow your arms to move forward and your hips to sit back.

Linear Lunge

(TONES THE THIGH MUSCLES)

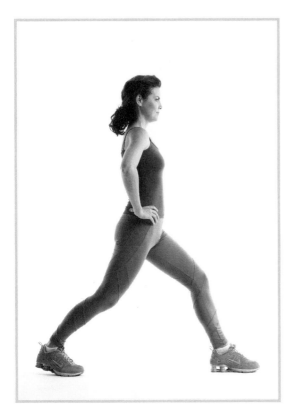

Stand tall with left foot approximately four feet in front of the right foot. Torso is upright and hands are comfortable at the waist.

Now simply bend both knees down, then straighten them both back up. Repeat ten times, then switch legs and perform ten more.

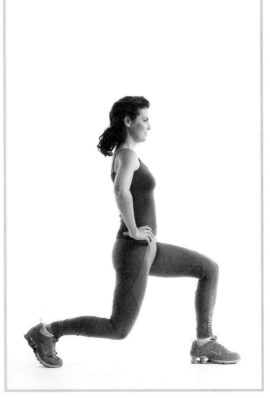

Perfect Push-Up

(TONES THE UPPER BODY)

Begin in Plank pose, with hands placed directly underneath the shoulder heads. Legs are straight.

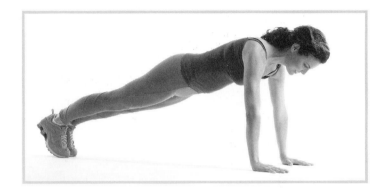

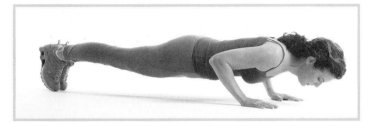

Inhale and bend both elbows, exhale and return back to the top. Repeat ten times total.

The Traditional Crunch

(SCULPTS THE ABDOMINAL MUSCLES)

Lie on your back with both knees bent and hands behind the head. Exhale and lift shoulder blades up off the floor. Inhale and return head and shoulders back down to the floor. Repeat twenty times total.

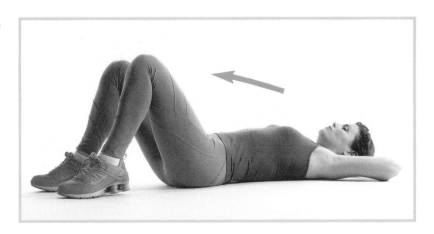

Side Curl

(HELPS TO TIGHTEN AND TONE THE WAISTLINE)

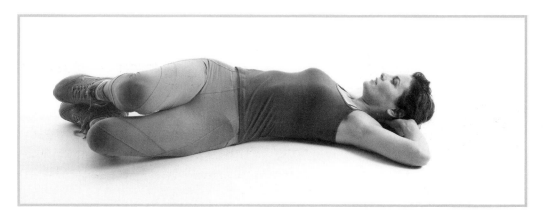

Lie on your back with both knees bent and folded to the left side. Hands are behind the head.

Exhale and lift shoulders up off the floor. Inhale and return back down. Do twenty repetitions, then drop the knees to the other side and perform twenty more.

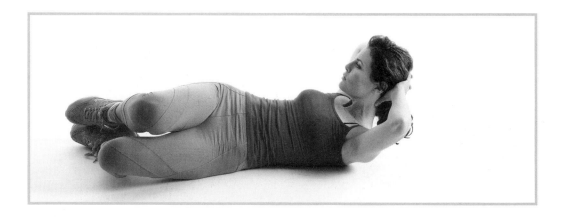

STEP 3: Standing Stretches. You spend enough time sitting on your butt, Taurus, so during your stretch section, you'll be upright, 100 percent. The last component of the Taurus workout is strategic standing stretches. Spend a full minute on each stretch.

Hamstring Stretch

(HELPS IMPROVE FLEXIBILITY IN THE HAMSTRINGS)

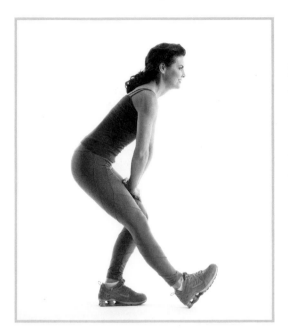

Stand with one foot approximately two feet in front of the other. Bend the rear knee, setting the hips back. Be sure to keep the front leg straight. You should feel a good stretch up the back of the thigh. Hold for sixty seconds, and then repeat on the other side.

Inner Thigh Stretch

(HELPS IMPROVE FLEXIBILITY IN THE INNER THIGH MUSCLES)

Stand with feet approximately three or four feet apart, toes pointing straight ahead. Lunge to the left and extend the right leg. Hold for sixty seconds, then switch the lunge to the right.

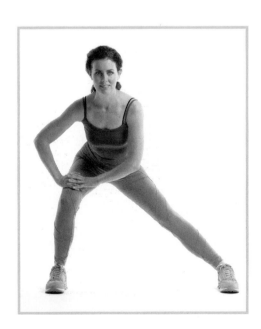

Balance Quad Stretch

(PROMOTES BETTER OVERALL BALANCE AND ALSO PROMOTES BETTER FLEXIBILITY IN THE QUADRICEPS. QUITE POSSIBLY YOUR TIGHTEST AREA!)

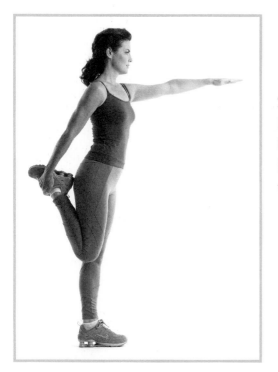

Stand on your left leg bending the right knee, hold the right foot with the right hand and bring the right heel toward the body. Use the left arm for balance. Hold for sixty seconds, then switch to the other side.

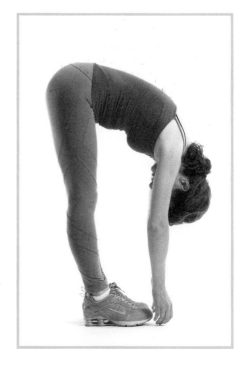

Spine Roll

(DE-STRESSES THE MUSCLES SURROUNDING THE SPINE)

Stand with feet in a parallel position. Smoothly and slowly roll your spine down to a forward bend position. Keep your eyes open at all times. Hold for sixty seconds and then roll up.

What's Ahead of Taurus: A Star-Driven Five-Year Plan

2007 This is your year for change! You can do anything you want to do, so if it's high time for you to run that marathon, go for it. You have the power, energy, and talent to achieve any goal; just make sure you have a few in mind.

Key Workout: Take up spinning or rock climbing, any cardio you admire but have not tried.

2008 It's a lucky year of power and steady-as-she-goes success. Your energy and health are unflagging. You look and feel great, so don't shy away from skintight activewear and enjoy being so busy you don't have time to overeat.

Key Workout: Travel somewhere new and go snowboarding, snorkeling, or rafting. Be in nature—you're a natural.

2009 Career focus can take your eyes off your active time. Hard work has a way of making it easy to have an extra margarita or one too many pasta dinners. Take the stress off by getting into fun. Walk with a chum so you can unload your anxiety and get some perspective on how life is not about getting the best of someone else.

Key Workout: Easygoing ambles or hikes with a massage at the end.

2010 You're going to feel the pressure to achieve something new. Accomplishing your goals will take hard work and determination; the stars will not let you be a quitter so buckle down and go for it.

Key Workout: Achievement-oriented goals. Acceleration, mileage, increased strength.

2011 This year's all about resistance. Resist the inner voice urging you to off-road nutrition and gorge. Resist self-criticism; resist the call of the couch. Resist giving up. Use this year's big surge of psychic energy to quietly create an amazing 180-degree transformation. Focus. That's all you need. (OK, that and resistance.)

Key Workout: One tight day-to-day plan that says you're in control.

zodiaction

Signs of Life

Taurus is not the only sign that influences your life. Look closely and openly at your love life and your career and you'll see people from different signs constantly appearing. You can read about them in this book so you know what makes them tick. Also, if you want to know more about what sign rules different parts of your life, check out these:

Love life—Scorpio

Career—Aquarius

Flirtation—Virgo

Health—Libra

gemini-action

THE TWINS May 21–June 20

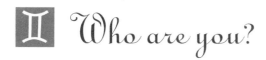

In One Word: CURIOUS

Symbol(s): The Twins. The Yin and the Yang. You are two sides of a whole. Remember the "half moon" cookie? That's you, light and dark.

Color: Silver (as in "quicksilver" and mercury)

Element: AIR. This is the realm of ideas, concepts, knowledge (as in gossip!), humor, and basic smarts. Air is hard to pin down and nice to have around—that is, when you're fresh. Air can also be foggy, smoggy, and stale, which happens when you're not stimulated or are feeling a bit stressed out. As an air sign you think, speak, and write before you feel things through. Sometimes air blows people off. Since air floats around us, you're not exactly grounded. It's a challenge for air signs to settle down into their bodies. But that's how you'll feel most effective when you put those amazing ideas to good use. So give up whisking around once in a while.

Energy: MUTABLE. You can bend, stretch, and do U-turns. Mutable energy is awesome for exercise since you're always moving and willing to try something new. But . . . how's that attention span? Mutable air signs are hard to pin down. One minute, you're an ardent fan of kickboxing and the next you're off to Hot Yoga. Get used to the fact that mutable can be inconsistent—but never boring or BORED.

zodiaction

Psychic Domain: Gemini rules communications, siblings, chatter, and wit. You can't stand slow-talkers, long explanations, or tedious topics. Gemini is about eloquence, resourcefulness, tolerance, and generosity. Your fitness plan must be dynamic, interesting, and changeable to suit your mood.

Physical Domain: Gemini rules the lungs, shoulders, arms, wrists, and hands. Nervous or anxious energy will settle on your shoulders (ouch), elbows, or even in your lungs and throat. Geminis like to run and walk, and swinging arms are helpful to open up your chest. If your upper back hurts or if you're having breathing problems, you are stressed out. That can be a sign to slow down and just find your center.

What to Avoid in the Gemini Workout: Monotonous exercise or anything that gives you a chance to get bored and quit.

Ideal Workout: Interesting, changeable workouts that give consistent results. Here's the thing: you want cardio that doesn't bore you, strength training that doesn't take what seems like a year in the gym, and flexibility work that you don't notice. And you want it to work really, really well or you'll quit. The right routine is no routine at all. You get choices and you even get a cop-out strategy for when you need to shake things up. And if you can talk on your cell phone, all the better.

Essential Workout Gear: Stretchy clothes, iPod.

Ultimate Trouble Spot: Lung capacity. And just to exacerbate the potential weakness, Gemini is also a sign that likes to smoke, especially when the naughty twin is in control.

Workout Buddy Warning: You need someone to talk to or no one at all. This has a lot to do with whether you're in the mood. If you do work out with someone, she can't be super-competitive and has to be able to persuade you to finish the whole workout.

If You Have a Personal Trainer:

1. Gemini's personal trainer must be interesting (and interested in you) and willing to talk about life outside of fitness.

2. Your trainer needs to shake things up A LOT, and send you on your way with varied routines you can do on your own.

3. Your trainer needs to be lax on the cancellation/rescheduling policy.

Strategic Choices for Gemini

The Gemini Diet: As a mutable sign, Gemini has different needs at different times, but you always need water, the element that is perhaps most easily ignored. It's cleansing, balancing, and mentally energizing, which can add much needed clarity when you're going in twelve directions at once. You also talk a lot, and water is the ideal drink to wet your palate, keeping your voice fresh. Since you have so much natural energy, you ~~don't need~~ **should not have** coffee or stimulants of any kind. (Just say no to Red Bull.) Now, we know you like a good buzz, but when your body is well-rested, well-watered, and well-fed, Gemini possesses a stellar natural high that exercise—and some juicy gossip—enhances.

You, The Twins, should also stay far, far away from candy. You have a very childlike attraction to all things bright, colorful, sugary, and seemingly exciting— *Sour Patch Kids, Jelly Bellies, Twizzlers, giant gumballs*—but these are extremely hazardous to a Gemini. Your Mercury influence makes your blood sugar levels surge and crash at lightning speed, taking your mind and spirit along for the roller-coaster ride.

Staying slim is a cinch for Gemini if you employ one basic technique: no eating on the run. As simple as it sounds, this is tough for a Gemini; you love to do more than one thing at once, after all, and multitasking is your forte. Don't eat and drive. Don't eat and walk. Don't eat and talk on the phone or enter a chat room. Don't eat and watch TV. Don't eat and read (especially gossip magazines and tabloids). When you eat, just eat. You're the perfect example of someone who thrives on eating five preplanned, small meals a day.

THE TOP THREE ITEMS TO SHOP FOR:

1. **Whole grain cereal in bulk.** No cereal bars, sports bars, or candy bars, which tend to be filled with artificial, overly processed ingredients; plus, they abet the Gemini crime of eating on the run.

2. **Bottled water and organic decaffeinated green tea.** You need to stay hydrated and warm.

3. **"Fun" fruit like kiwi, mangos, and watermelon.** Unusual, colorful, and seasonal fruit can fulfill your candy desires and be good for you at the same time.

Diet Vice: Candy.
Signature Spa Treatment: Aromatherapy.
Complementary Therapy: Guided meditations.
Mindfulness Mantra: If I focus, I'll know what I need to know.

Gemini is the know-it-all, chatterbox, and gossip correspondent of the zodiac. The Gemini needs mental stimulation at all times—and that's not so hard since you're interested in so many things. While the search and seizure of knowledge and witticisms are fine for free time, the key to Gemini wisdom is in sitting still and turning off your mind. It's a lifelong karmic challenge but you are best when rested, focused, and able to access the deep wells of knowledge you possess through your intuitive and intellectual capacity. That means sit down, shut up, and silence your mind. Meditate. You need the space to settle down, know what you know, and find your center, then get up again and shake up the world one story at a time. You really don't need to get to know every person you meet, and learning to screen will be helpful. Your health and fitness are largely dependent on how much time you leave for yourself. So, you're your own worst enemy and your own best friend, depending on which Twin is in charge.

Gemini in a Nutshell

MIND: Sharper than a tack, faster than a speeding bullet, the centerpiece of your fabulousness is all about your head and what's in it. Your self-esteem sinks when you think you don't know the answer. Your mind is where you're most comfortable. But if you spend all your time there, when will you play, love, and live? Give your head a rest once in a while and see what it's like to just feel.

BODY: Gemini has a quick, agile body and the ability to use it productively. But you're not exactly paying attention to it when you're talking or running off to meet friends. You're apt to be too busy to care about food and go for the easy fix. You might blow off an exercise class or even a doctor's appointment when there's something more interesting to do. Do you need to be told that's not so good? The more you respect your body, the better you'll feel, the clearer your mind—and you know that's what it's all about.

SPIRIT: You connect people and thoughts with your airy, vibrant energy. You light up circuits of knowledge in the world without judgment.

Stay clear so that your connections are strong and your knowledge is pure. Take time to listen so you can share what you hear.

Two Gemini Workout Stories (Two for The Twins)

BARRIE

I grew up in a family whose motto was "If you feel the urge to exercise, lie down until it passes." I loved getting exercise though, and once I got to college I took modern dance, lifted weights, and swam laps. Then I started to run and play tennis. When I started working in New York I joined a health club, took aerobics, used a personal trainer occasionally, got into Step class, but not spinning (why ride a bike that goes nowhere?), then went back to swimming laps. And running. And then I took classes again. This year I'm into walking, doing Ellen's routines, and some body sculpting. Last year I took classes and swam. Consistent? Absolutely. I always get exercise. Routine? Nah. Too boring.

ELLEN

I'm a classic Gemini—very enthusiastic and curious about the latest and greatest. Over the years, I've gleefully gone through every workout craze you can think of: aerobics, Jazzercise, Step, spinning, Tae-Bo, yoga, and Pilates. I've loved them all, and then kicked 'em to the curb. My Rollerblades fell to their death in 1995, one week after their purchase. I coveted them for a few sunny afternoons of "blading" with my girlfriends, then poof! Off to the attic they went, never to be seen again.

I don't officially have Attention Deficit Disorder (ADD), but my Gemini ways sure make me seem ADD-*ish* and there is no way around it—it's written in the stars.

zodiaction

My eyes are blue, my attention is fleeting, and that's my reality. Nothing exercise-related held my interest until I discovered *fusion fitness,* where the mind and body are trained together, the variety is endless, and the results are quick. *Fusion fitness* is a term used for a form of exercise that blends two or more different disciplines. I figure I'll be sixty before I've exhausted all of the possibilities. Could anything be more perfect for Gemini?

THE GEMINI "MULTITASKER" WORKOUT

A successful Gemini workout has three parts: 1. A cardio/sculpt *Ballerina Cardio* section appeals to the Gemini multitasking spirit and her need for a faster pace. 2. A stretch/strength *Power Barre* section appeals again to the multitasker Twin, but also demands a mind–body connection. 3. The Gemini workout finishes with a simple chill-out exercise, which is ultra-soothing for the Gemini nervous system, which seemingly gets short-circuited easier than the other signs.

THREE WORKOUT GOALS FOR GEMINI

1. Avoid getting bored by inserting variety into the routine.

- Do the same exercises in a different order.

- Change up the music. (We think the iPod was invented specifically for Geminis.)

- Invite different people to work out with you.

- Add ankle/wrist weights to your routine.

2. Finish what you start. Do every exercise. Do every rep. Dig deep for discipline.

3. Make a mind–body connection right from the start. Gemini tends to drift off into la-la land when the mind isn't paying attention to the goings-on of the workout.

WORKOUT PRESCRIPTION

Find something that interests you and try it out. If you don't like it, move on. If you love it, stick to it until you don't. The biggest Gemini workout trap is to feel like you can't make a change. You don't even have to commit to a routine. If you're into running today, go for it. If you'd rather take a yoga class, fine. Listen to your energy, your mood, and your body.

There is no shame in walking on a treadmill and watching TV, or riding a stationary bike and reading a book. If that helps you exercise, do it. Your iPod is your BFF, as is your cell phone (but watch where you are when you jabber away).

BEST TIME TO WORK OUT: Anytime! Variety is your spice of life.

STEP 1: Ballerina Cardio (three in one! strength, cardio, and poise). Three exercises:

Traveling Plié

(EXCELLENT EXERCISE FOR SCULPTING LEANER-LOOKING THIGHS)

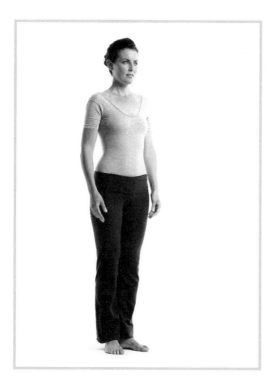
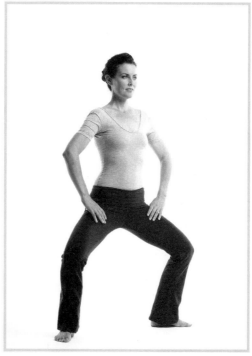

Stand tall with heels together and toes slightly turned out.

Keep your torso completely vertical, step out to the right, and, as you do so, bend both knees. Then squeeze the muscles of your legs and butt as you return to the starting position. Repeat twenty times total, alternating right and left, at a brisk up-tempo pace.

Alternating Arabesque

(A BEAUTIFUL EXERCISE THAT PROMOTES BETTER BALANCE AND POSTURE)

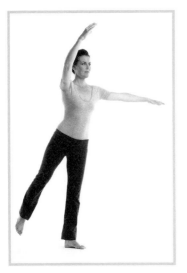 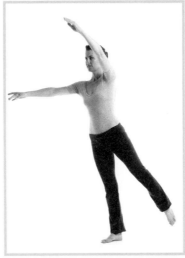

Stand on your straight right leg with right arm extended upward toward the ceiling, left leg lifted slightly behind you, abs in, and shoulders down.

Kick back with your left leg (feel a "lift" in your butt cheek), then in one graceful move, switch to the other side, planting the left leg and lifting the left arm up. Repeat twenty times, alternating right and left, at a brisk up-tempo pace.

Dancer Lunge

(TONES THE BUTTOCKS AND THIGHS)

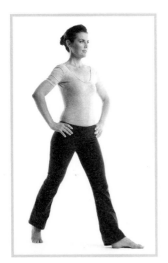 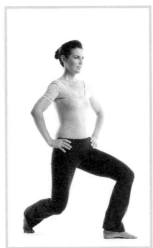

Stand with both feet turned out slightly and with the left foot approximately four feet in front of the right.

Simply bend both knees simultaneously, keeping the torso vertical. Return smoothly back up to the starting position. Repeat ten times with left leg forward, then ten more times with the right leg forward, for a total of twenty.

STEP 2: Power Barre—or Chair Back (stretch and strengthen the muscles of the body simultaneously). Five exercises:

Tiptoe One-Legged Bend

(SIMULTANEOUSLY STRETCHES AND STRENGTHENS JUST ABOUT EVERY MUSCLE IN THE LEG)

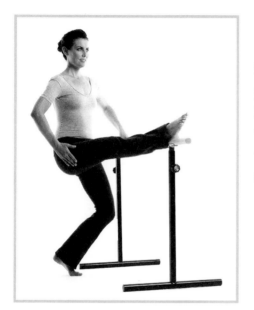

Stand on the left leg in a relevé or "tiptoe" position. Place the right leg on the barre. Keep the torso tall and lifted. Now, on your tiptoes, simply bend the left knee and hold for thirty seconds. Be sure to repeat on the other leg.

Side Stretch

(SIMULTANEOUSLY STRETCHES AND STRENGTHENS JUST ABOUT EVERY MUSCLE IN THE LEG)

Place the left leg, extended, on the barre and reach the right arm up and over toward the barre. Hold for sixty seconds. You want to feel the side body and leg muscles simultaneously stretch and squeeze. Repeat on the other side.

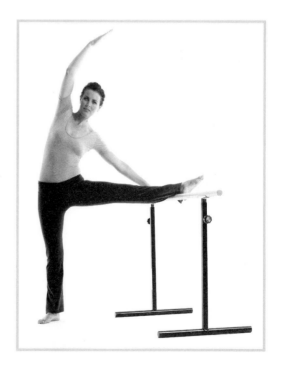

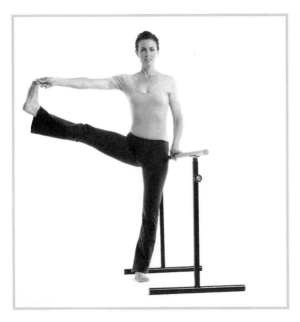

Leg Extension

(STRETCHES THE INNER THIGH AND IMPROVES THE RANGE OF MOTION IN THE HIPS)

Standing adjacent to the barre, lightly hold on to it with your left hand. With your right hand, grab hold of your right foot and extend it up to hip level (or higher). Try to keep the knee completely straight. This is to be held for sixty seconds. You want to notice the side body and leg muscles simultaneously stretch and squeeze providing amazing toning effects. Repeat on the other side.

Isolation Butt Squeeze

(A VERY EFFECTIVE EXERCISE FOR TIGHTENING THE BUTTOCK MUSCLES)

Stand tall, with your ears stacked upon the shoulders, shoulders stacked upon the hips, adjacent to the barre in first position (heels together, toes slightly turned out). Bend both knees and lift up both heels. This is the starting position. The knees stay bent and the heels stay lifted throughout the entire exercise. Now, exhale and scoop the belly and press the pelvis forward, squeezing all of the butt muscles. Return to starting position on an inhalation. Repeat twenty times total.

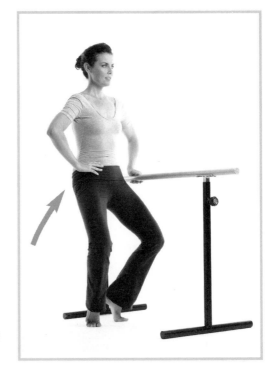

Bow-Pulling Squeeze

*(THIS IS NOT A POSE, BUT AN ACTUAL REPETITION EXERCISE
THAT DE-STRESSES THE ENTIRE FRONT BODY, CREATING LONGER-LOOKING BODYLINES.)*

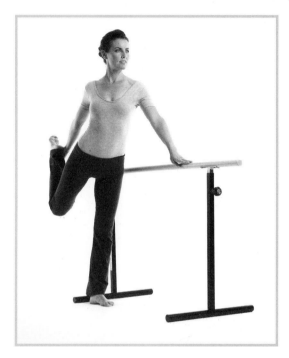

Stand tall, adjacent to the barre. Hold the barre lightly with your left hand and hold your right ankle with your right hand.

Inhale and kick right foot back, all the while keeping it in the right hand. Mindfully, slide the left hand forward on the barre. You should feel an incredible stretching feeling in the entire front body. Exhale and return to the starting position. Repeat ten times, switch sides and repeat ten more.

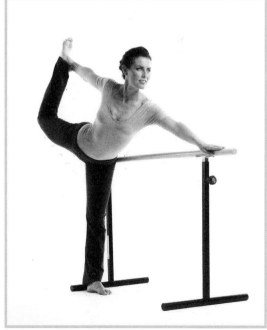

STEP 3: Chill Out (soothe the nervous system by inverting the legs). One exercise:

Legs up the Wall

(THIS EXERCISE HELPS REJUVENATE TIRED LEGS)

Kick off your shoes and bring your body to any clear wall. Extend both legs straight up the wall, with your head, shoulders, and back completely resting on the ground. Ideally, the body forms a 90-degree "L" angle. Hold for anywhere between sixty seconds and five minutes.

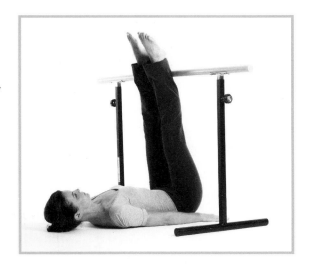

What's Ahead of Gemini: A Star-Driven Five-Year Plan

2007   This is a year you're going to want a workout buddy. Partnership issues are highlighted and your head is turning every time someone cute passes you by. It's ideal for getting along with people and forming lasting friendships—maybe try training for a marathon—it's more fun with someone to celebrate with. **Key Workout:** Social opportunities like running outside, tennis doubles, or golf (only if you walk).

2008   Planetary pressures can instigate sweeping changes. This is great fun when you're up for something new but tough when you're tired. Since you can't control the outside world, you can only work with how you react to it. Workouts need to leave you refreshed, enlivened, and calm. **Key Workout:** Walking with your iPod, fat-burning stretch and strengthen classes, swimming slow laps.

2009   If you can't find your inner focus, it's because you left it at a cocktail party. That's sort of what this year is like. You're on an experiential rampage. If you haven't tried it, you will, probably with someone who is an expert, who will take good care of you, and who has a totally dreamy gaze.
Key Workout: Extreme skiing, alpine hiking, Habitat for Humanity.

2010   Being busy is no excuse and being successful is even more reason to stick to your fitness plans. It's all about accomplishment and being rewarded for work well done. So put some effort into yourself too, and see what great shape really means.
Key Workout: Goal-oriented workouts with action, inspiration, and flexible timing. At-home DVDs?

2011   In an unusual year for Gemini, you're almost ready to turn off the phone. There is a certain amount of planetary overload that could push your energy right off the nervous edge. Burning fat is easy, so give yourself the time to do less strenuous workouts that concentrate on grounding, centering your energy, and restoring sanity.
Key Workout: Hot Yoga, silent walking, swimming laps.

Signs of Life

Gemini, like all signs, has a lot more astrological influence than just the surface. As The Twins, you are always exploring life in all its aspects. But you're not so Gemini when it comes to your love life, your work, or your health. Ever wonder why you're kind of spacey at work? Or why you're an extremist when it comes to your body? Read up on these signs and get more insight into yourself and all your fascinating Gemini facets!

Love life—Sagittarius

Career—Pisces

Flirtation—Libra

Health—Scorpio

cancer-action

THE CRAB June 21–July 22

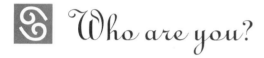 *Who are you?*

In One Word: SENSITIVE

Symbol(s): The Crab. You carry your house on your back. Cautious, kind, tenacious, and loyal, you are the nurturer-mother of the zodiac. You take careful, sideways steps but you get where you want to go.

Color: Shimmering silver

Element: WATER. Cancer is the first water sign of the zodiac. Most of the time, water conducts energy which makes you very perceptive to others' feelings. You feel deeply, sometimes in a flood of emotions. In that case, you use your shell to protect yourself from being too open. Hard on the outside, soft on the inside, you're the Tootsie Roll Pop of the zodiac but you're not always sweet! When you're forced to fight, you have very effective claws. And when you're happy, you're floating on warm waves of love. Being a water sign is tremendously psychic, but you have to learn how to keep your water clear and pure. Don't get bogged down by the sludge from earth.

Energy: CARDINAL. Like Aries, you like a single, targeted goal and you'll get there without a problem. It might take you some time to achieve what you want, though, since Crabs do prefer to sidle rather than to sprint. You stubbornly commit to a path and once you set out, it takes three times the effort to make a change. Fortunately, you're not likely to "go for it" without a lot of thought and consideration. Average cardinal water signs do well in swim aerobics classes because you're in your element and you don't have to decide what to do. Motivated Cancer girls, however, are great athletes: persistent, patient, and achieving.

Psychic Domain: Cancers rule the nurturing inner voice, intuition, and mother-wisdom. You certainly don't have to have children to access this knowledge—you possess a psychic heritage that accompanies you throughout your life. Cancer is about making choices based on your heart. When you're bogged down with negativity you'll crawl into your shell. The irony is that feeling better comes from the love of others, and being exposed enough to feel it. Ruled by the moon, Cancers are very tied to moon cycles. Waxing moons are building energy, waning moons are decreasing energy. Full moons are "anything goes."

Physical Domain: Cancer rules the stomach, skin, and breasts. Being stressed out is basically a stomachache or an acne breakout when you're a Cancer. You are very sensitive to impurities—even emotional "dirt"—so your body will tell you right away if something is wrong. It's great to sweat it out while swimming, running, hiking, doing any kind of aerobic activity, especially followed by a sauna or steam. You're constantly taking in more vibes than you need so feel free to sweat it out. It can keep your skin clear too.

What to Avoid in the Cancer Workout: Crawling into your shell and forgetting to exercise.

Ideal Workout: You are not fragile, just sensitive, so you can take a tough workout as long as it is presented in a very fluid, non-intimidating way. Your workouts also vary depending on your mood. When you're calm and happy, go for a bike ride, or take the dog to the park. When you get crabby, instead of pulling into that shell, seek solitude in exercise, perhaps with a solo run or a non-partner yoga session. Swimming, of course, is natural for you, but could be tough on your skin. You'll also be highly motivated with any "Walk for the Cure" or fund-raising race that's dear to your heart. You are quick to say yes when helping others is involved.

Essential Workout Gear: A soft, easy, nonrestrictive sweat suit.

Ultimate Trouble Spot: Abs.

Workout Buddy Warning: Your workout buddy has to possess two qualities: She must not be competitive (No "I'll race you to the stop sign" antics!). And she should be on the quieter side. A nonstop talker is overwhelming for The Crab.

If You Have a Personal Trainer:

1. Look for yoga-types, who tend to be more telepathic and better equipped to feel your mood.

2. Ideally, this trainer comes to you. Go ahead; pay the extra cash for PT house calls.

3. Male trainers can be more forthright. They tend to be less invasive when it comes to your inner radar.

Strategic Choices for Cancer

The Cancer Diet: As a water sign, you are keenly aware of the fact that your body is four-fifths water. Your challenge is to keep yourself in a state of equilibrium by staying away from too much water (hello, bloat) and too little water (constipation, anyone?). You know when you're in balance because your skin glows, your tummy is flat, and you flow through your life with easy energy. You know when your waters are running poorly too. That's when toxins easily take over your complexion and you notice dry, spotty, or ruddy skin. To get rid of excess water, diluted cranberry juice and herbal teas are your friends. To gather more water into your system, try having oatmeal for breakfast. But instead of adding brown sugar, squeeze some 100-percent-pure maple syrup into your bowl and stir. It's better for your complexion because it isn't processed.

Greasy foods are bad for every sign, but they are Cancer's enemy #1, exacerbating every one of your negative tendencies—they're hard to digest, bad for your arteries, and put you into a crabby mental state. Salty foods may seem irresistible to you—Crabs are saltwater creatures after all—but don't give in to your cravings all the time. And if you add salt to dishes, make it sea salt, which, because it has higher mineral content, will integrate into your meals more gracefully than processed table salt. Also try spicing things up with paprika, cayenne pepper, or ginger if needed. These spices help circulation and have no sodium. Also beware that water signs are particularly vulnerable to alcohol. It doesn't take much to get you tipsy.

To stick to a decent diet, you need to eat at home as much as possible. You'll have less difficulty following this through because, let's face it, Cancer girls are homebodies. You like to control your environment and your atmosphere, so it's just healthier, in mind, body, and spirit, when you prepare your own meals. And, wow, you actually enjoy grocery shopping. Cancer finds great comfort in stocked cupboards and overflowing freezers. You'll also be more aware of what you're eating and that's exactly what you need to lose or maintain your weight. You can't resist a bag of salty chips once in a while—so don't. Just flush with water and return to better choices when you're over that craving.

Cancer might just be the queen of the kitchen. The Crab can cook! You are apt to use healthy ingredients too, so we don't have to preach to you about partially hydrogenated oil and animal fats, but we must warn you about one thing: PORTION CONTROL. Use a salad plate for your entrée, fill it up, and don't go back for seconds. You don't want to be a stuffed crab, do you? So what to do with the leftovers? Put them in that fancy Tupperware of yours, in individual portions. Send one container next door to your widowed neighbor (she loves your cuisine!) and put the rest in your freezer.

THE TOP THREE ITEMS TO SHOP FOR:

1. **Gourmet sea salts.** Splurge on different varieties.

2. **Extra virgin olive oil.** Good for cooking, and good for your skin.

3. **Pellegrino.** Instead of wine with dinner (remember, alcohol really wreaks havoc on The Crab), have a glass of Pellegrino. Sip it from a water goblet too, for extra elegance.

Diet Vice: Volume—watch out for too much of anything.

Signature Spa Treatment: Mineral bath.

Complementary Therapy: Salt scrub.

Mindfulness Mantra: My emotions are my reality and reality provides me with infinite love.

Cancer is the mother of the zodiac, the nurturer, the feminine mystery maiden. Tough on the outside, soft on the inside, you demand honesty, loyalty, and love from your friends and family and you give only the best in return. When you lose yourself in a relationship, sometimes "mothering" becomes "smothering." Knowing when to back off is important, otherwise you'll feel hurt and retreat into your shell. You can do anything—ANYTHING—when you focus on a goal. You're smart and you take your time, get comfortable with your situation, then make progress, sure, and steady. The Crab isn't a gusto-grabbing spotlight-hogger. You're the one who quietly attracts a fan base and then moves organically along with a large support group. You can be the star if you want to be, but your real joy comes from just being with the people you love. Of course, the world is full of new people and experiences, and even though you can be shy, you must learn to adjust to new situations. When you turn on the charm, there's no one better to be around. But when you're overtired or you don't like someone, it's not that easy to cover it up. Stay rested, stay confident in yourself, and you won't be uncomfortable or crabby—and that's your key to happiness.

Cancer in a Nutshell

MIND: Cancers have a great memory, especially for the times you've been hurt or wronged. If you can let go of the grudges embedded in your mind, you'll be open to a whole lot more good stuff. You already know a lot but it doesn't start in your head. Your intuition is stronger than your other senses and you have access to great wisdom. When you do need to think something through, take it into your heart. That's where your answers are.

BODY: You're not built for speed or competition, but you're athletic when you're interested. Your physical body is soothing to others, warm, comforting, and quietly sexy. Cancer has a soft, lovely feminine form but can get skin or stomach troubles from being off balance. Instead of reaching for the covers or resting on the couch when you're feeling unhealthy or unpresentable, make sure you get out into the elements. Water needs some air now and then.

SPIRIT: You are the deepest feminine love and power. You share it with those who respect it and you show it to those who need to learn from it.

Flow freely with your feelings and feel the strength of their power.
Let yourself be vulnerable so others can give you strength.

zodiaction

A Cancer Workout Story

Rachel got into the best shape of her life when she hired Tony to be her personal trainer. She worked hard, lost fifteen pounds, and her mood was a steady flow of happiness. Her abs were tight and she fit into her favorite pair of jeans for the first time in years. Then one day, Tony had a "family emergency" and passed Rachel off to his fellow trainer, Bruce. Apparently Tony told Bruce about a few of Rachel's idiosyncrasies, like how she liked to train in the more private corner on the second floor and how her brow perspiration was epic and she thus needed a towel around her neck—ready to go—at all times. This felt like an invasion of privacy to Rachel. After her hour-long one-on-one session with Bruce, she retreated home in a crabby state, upset that Tony divulged such seemingly intimate information about her. After a few days of hiding in her shell, Rachel emerged to phone Tony to cancel her standing weekly appointment. She didn't give Tony any specific reason, just saying that "She wasn't feeling up to working out today." Rachel never went back to Tony, even though he had worked her into A+ shape. In fact, Rachel never again hired a personal trainer.

One-on-one personal training, like a doctor's appointment, is intimate. Every relationship involving Cancer depends on bona fide trust right from the start. This is a classic Cancer scenario of trust. Trust is vital, yet fleeting, to The Crab. One wrong move and Wham! The trust is lost.

THE CANCER "POWER FLOW" WORKOUT

A successful Cancer workout starts off with a very thorough stretch section that targets the upper, middle, and lower back areas. It parlays into just a touch of strength training for enhancing posture, and then finishes with fluid cardio such as swimming, the NordicTrack, and walking/jogging to a consistent beat. It is of paramount importance that Cancer avoid the gym by working out at home or outdoors whenever possible. Cancers aren't gym types. You get too easily irritated by the dumbbell-lifting grunters and the cell phone talkers. Plus, you tend to be more self-conscious than many of the other astrological signs, making the gym—especially the coed kind—a scary place. The Crab dislikes handheld weights or cumbersome equipment, preferring more freedom in movement. Cancer is also against blatant abs work, unlike Virgo, who wants to target the core all day long! We'll disguise crunches and sit-ups; by inserting some abdominal focus in the cardio section you won't even realize we're toning your belly.

THREE WORKOUT GOALS FOR CANCER—ALL TIED TO THE MOON

Cancer, being ruled by the moon, is extra sensitive to lunar positioning. (Let the moon be your personal trainer!)

1. Use the waxing moon for building endurance and strength (when the moon goes from new to full).

2. Use the waning moon to develop flexibility and stamina.

3. Use the full moon to do something new.

WORKOUT PRESCRIPTION

Work with your energy, not against it. You can consult your local paper or the Internet to find out what stage the moon is in. You'll notice that your energy goes up as the moon works toward the full moon. Once that moon is full, your energy will peak and then slowly wane. Although every sign can feel the effects of the moon's energy as it shifts into new phases, you are particularly sensitive. If you try to push yourself just before the moon is new (this is called an "old moon") you'll feel very tired. Better to learn the moon's phases and let natural forces guide you through the month. Your energy has a high tide and low tide and we do not want you to get beached!

BEST TIME TO WORK OUT: Evening.

STEP 1: The Elite Eight Stretch Series. Stretching comes first for you, Cancer. It'll calm your psyche, and prepare your body for more strenuous movement. The key to remember with *The Elite Eight Stretch Series* is this: **stretch with vigor.** These are not "chill-out stretches"—notice you are never resting on your back—they are aggressive stretches, where you hold positions for sixty seconds each with muscular energy.

Lots of attention is paid to The Crab's back, moving it every which way. Tightness tends to migrate into your spine, causing stiffness and limited range of motion. Here we loosen up those tension pockets, creating better fluidity in movement.

Cat Stretch

(STRETCHES UPPER CHEST, MAKING BREATHING EASIER AND MOVING ENERGY THROUGHOUT THE SPINE)

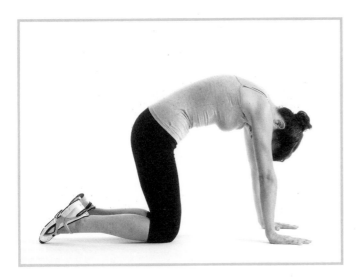

Position yourself on your hands and knees. The knees should line up directly underneath your hips and hands should be placed directly underneath the heads of the shoulders. Round your back, by pressing the navel up toward the spine, tucking your tailbone underneath the hips, and pointing the crown of the head toward the floor. Hold for sixty seconds, then release.

Cow Stretch

(STRETCHES ALL OF THE MUSCLES OF THE BACK AND GETS ENERGY MOVING THROUGHOUT THE SPINE)

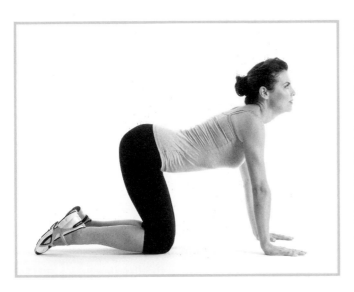

Position yourself on your hands and knees. The knees should line up directly underneath your hips and the hands should be placed directly underneath the heads of the shoulders. Arch your back by gazing up toward the ceiling, pointing your tailbone upward, and squeezing the shoulder blades together on your back. Hold for sixty seconds, then release.

Rhomboid Stretch

(DEEPLY STRETCHES THE MIDDLE-UPPER BACK, RELEASING OODLES OF TENSION)

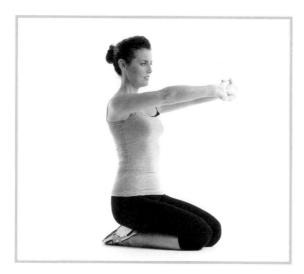

Kneel on the ground, stretch your arms out in front with fingers laced. Pull strongly, straightening both elbows, with a tension-releasing feeling in the mid-upper back. Bring your chin inward, toward the chest, and feel the shoulder blades open apart. Hold for sixty seconds, then release.

Ball Pose

(SUBTLY STRETCHES THE LOWER BACK, WHILE PULLING ON THE ABDOMINAL MUSCLES AND IMPROVING BALANCE)

This stretch is also called the *Pilates Balance Point.* Balance on your hips with both feet off the floor. Hold on to your lower leg (ideally the ankle) and round your back, forming a ball shape. Feel a great stretch in the lower back. Hold for sixty seconds, then release.

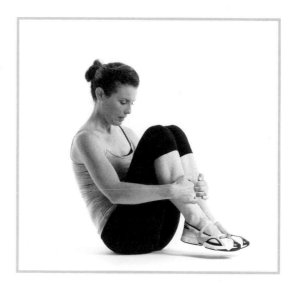

63

Runner's Stretch

(STRETCHES THE MUSCLES OF THE LEGS)

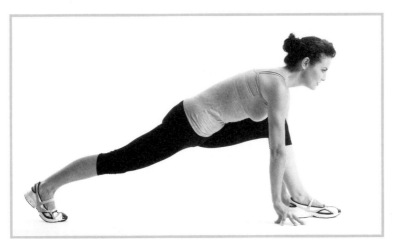

Lunge, with your left leg forward, and hands on either side of the left foot. Keep the right leg as extended as possible. The left knee should form a 90-degree angle with the floor. Hold for sixty seconds, then release and repeat with the right leg forward.

Straddle Stretch

(SIMULTANEOUSLY STRETCHES THE LOWER BACK AND THE HAMSTRING MUSCLES)

From a seated upright position, straddle both legs as wide as possible, keeping your knees straight. From this position, reach the left hand toward the outer right leg. Hold for sixty seconds, then release and repeat on the left leg.

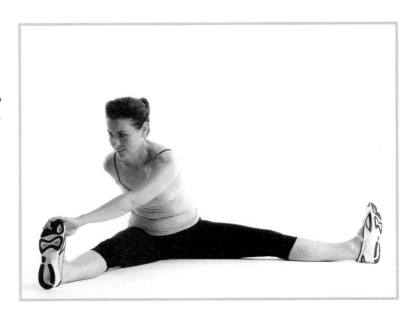

Ear-to-Shoulder Stretch

(RELEASES TENSION BUILDUP ALONG THE NECK SILHOUETTE)

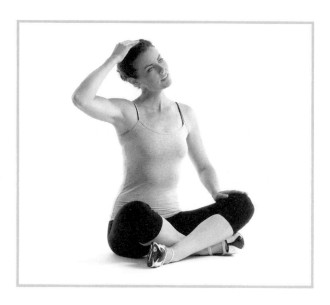

Sit on the floor, cross-legged with the spine upright, head straight atop the shoulders. Take the right hand to the head and lightly pull the head toward the right shoulder. Feel a nice stretch up the left side of the neck. Hold for sixty seconds, then release and repeat on the left.

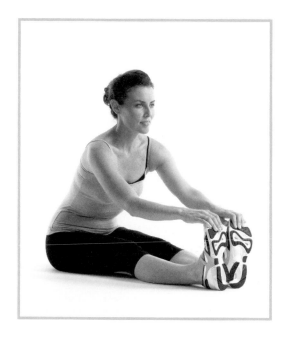

Seated Forward Bend

(SIMULTANEOUSLY AND DEEPLY STRETCHES THE LOWER BACK MUSCLES, HAMSTRINGS, AND CALVES)

From a sitting position, extend both legs out in front of you. Flex your feet and tilt your upper body forward, reaching for your lower legs or (preferably) your feet. Grab hold of either the legs or the feet for leverage. Pull the torso down toward the toes. Hold for sixty seconds, then release.

STEP 2: Side-Lying Strength Series. Crabs like to move laterally, so these side-lying exercises should be very appealing. Also we are developing strength here with no added equipment, for that awesome feeling of freedom Cancer loves.

Side Leg Lift

(TONES THE THIGH MUSCLES AND SIDE-WAIST MUSCLES EFFECTIVELY)

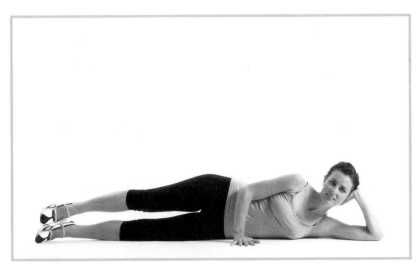

Lie on your side, forming a straight line. Lay your head in your bottom hand and place your top arm in front of you on the floor for support.

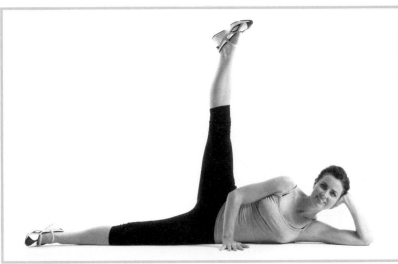

Point your toes, inhale, and lift the right leg straight up. Aim for a completely vertical bodyline at the height of the movement. Exhale and flex the foot, returning to the starting position. Repeat ten times, then release and perform the exact same number of repetitions on the other side.

Side Bend

(PERFECTLY TONES ALL OF THE MUSCLES OF THE CORE)

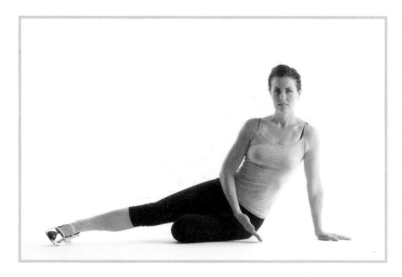

Begin by placing the left hand on the floor, directly below the shoulder head. Bend the left knee on the floor and extend the right leg. The hips are slightly up off the floor, so your body weight is being held by your limbs.

Inhale and reach the right arm up and overhead, taking the torso upward as well. Exhale and return to the starting position. Repeat ten times, then release and perform the exact same number of repetitions on the other side.

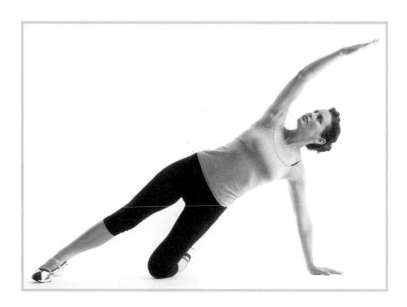

Knee Fold

(AN EXCELLENT STRENGTHENER FOR THE GLUTES, LOWER ABDOMINALS, AND OUTER THIGH MUSCLES)

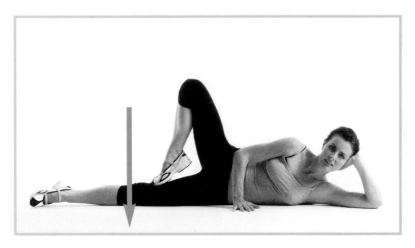

Begin by lying on your side and positioning the body in a long straight line. Prop the head up with the bottom hand and bend the top knee, resting the toes on the inner thigh. Exhale and fold the knee in front, aiming for the floor.

Try not to move anything else—just isolate the movement to the hip. Inhale and return to the starting position. Repeat ten times, then release and perform the exact same number of repetitions on the other side.

Inner Thigh Leg Beat

(ONE OF THE ALL-TIME GREATS FOR TONING THE CORE AND THE INNER THIGH SIMULTANEOUSLY)

Balance your torso on your forearm and hip. Extend both legs and raise them off the floor. Hinge slightly at the hip, forming a slight angle with the body. Point the feet and toes.

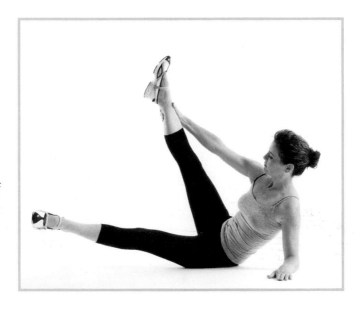

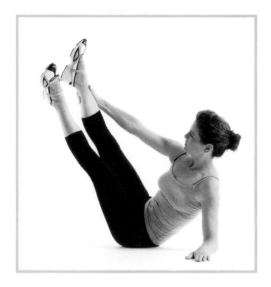

Exhale and lift the bottom leg up to meet the top leg. Inhale and return to the starting position. Repeat ten times, then release and perform the exact same number of repetitions on the other side.

STEP 3: Smooth Cardio with a Posture Emphasis. (Aim for thirty minutes in duration.) Cancer, we need you to break a sweat during cardio in order to release surface toxins. This means on a scale of one to ten (ten being the highest), Cancer's intensity should hover around 7.5 from beginning to end. The two other parts to the Cancer workout are not going to produce much perspiration, so we planned on your cardio component to do just that.

Cancer's cardio component is also last in sequence for two good reasons. One, the stretch and the strength sections have gracefully awakened your body—for you are not quick off the starting blocks! Two, the two prior sections have put you in a state of mind that is conducive to exercise. You are ready to come out of your shell for real.

Also, whether you choose for your cardio thirty minutes on the Elliptical machine, the StairMaster, or a jaunt outdoors, don't hunch over. Pull those shoulders back, lift your heart, and stand tall. Cancer must be aware of what's going on in the core. Stability, stability, stability. Here is where your abdominal focus comes into play. Engage your core by imagining you have a tight corset on. (You can actually wear a tightly fitting belt if you don't want to imagine!) This will not only make the cardio seem easier, it will tighten and tone your abdominal muscles as well.

zodiaction

What's Ahead of Cancer: A Star-Driven Five-Year Plan

2007   Welcome to the year of Healthy New You. The stars line up to give you solid energy, great vitality, and great goals to work for. You'll work hard this year and it only makes you stronger and more successful when you feel fit and feisty. Your input pays off so don't hesitate to really go for it.
Key Workout: Squash with a friend.

2008   Planets move into new signs and you might get tongue-tied when you hook up with major romance. Since you don't need words to express yourself, you can use body language. Ah, that requires some preparation. Make sure that when someone else's fingers do the walking they find smooth terrain.
Key Workout: Kundalini Yoga, African dancing.

2009   Sweeping changes aren't like you at all but this year you toy with the idea of breaking ground on new goals. Luck is on your side and, although you take it all very seriously, there will be fun behind that previously closed door. So open it up, take some risks (small risks), and see how happy you can get.
Key Workout: Cycling in preparation for a bicycle vacation with a cool new group.

2010   It's all about learning, seeking, and adventure. Sure, you can do this with a book or at a movie, but there's an itch that has to be scratched and it's called "Watch me!" Will you be diving off the high dive or just finding different ways to go down the Super Water Slide? It doesn't matter since you'll have fun and thrills either way.
Key Workout: Water aerobics or lap swimming.

2011   Planets are squaring off this year and that makes The Crab feisty and fussy. The good news is that your take-no-BS attitude goes over well at work. The not-so-good is that you'll want to hide in your shell until the urge to stand up for yourself passes. Honey, you haven't come this far to play dead. So get up, get on those gloves, and swing that punch. You're a knockout, remember?
Key Workout: Tae Kwon Do (a modern martial art from Korea that is characterized by its high kicks).

Signs of Life

Cancer has the propensity to crawl into a safe, warm place and shut out the world. Thankfully, you are not so easily hidden. Below are the other astrological signs that color your chart with different layers. In your career, you're a warrior. In your love life, you're dignified on the outside, a devil on the inside. Don't worry, we won't tell your secrets. But you know, it's worth sharing a little bit of yourself every now and then!

Love life–Capricorn

Career–Aries

Flirtation–Scorpio

Health–Sagittarius

leo-action

THE LION July 23—August 22

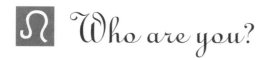

In One Word: REGAL

Symbol(s): The Lion. You are a born leader, a fearless protector, and one who appreciates being appreciated. Leo is the king of the zodiac, majestic, inspired, and generous. When your subjects don't please you, however, you can be arrogant and fussy.

Color: Majestic purple

Element: FIRE. As the second fire sign of the zodiac, you pick up from where Aries left off. You're not an independent firecracker; you're the sun. Your energy is the center of your own personal solar system. Leo fire lights up hearts and inspires others to join in, to play, and to make this world a better—and more fun—place. You bring amusements like sports, entertainment, and playful flirtation. Your energy shines a spotlight on those around you; however, some of us don't want to be in it. Leo fire needs to tone down sometimes just to take a look around and see who wants to play. For the most part you are dignified, amusing, and generous. But Leo fire is also self-involved. You need loyal subjects and playmates so watch how much time you spend gazing at your own image. Too much self-admiration and you might be attractive but you won't be popular.

zodiaction

Energy: FIXED. Leo is the second fixed sign of the zodiac, extra-strength in don't-tell-me-what-to-do energy than your fellow fixed sign Taurus. Exercise classes aren't for you unless you look really hot in your workout gear. Your Leo dignity, self-esteem, and vision might keep you from getting help with your fitness strategy, but—let's face it—even kings use advisors. Sometimes you need to move to the beat from someone else's drum. So channel fellow Leo Madonna and dance to music that makes you want to move.

Psychic Domain: Leos rule benevolent generosity and rarely suffer from big self-esteem issues. You are lionhearted, happy to use your inborn influence and kindness to help those in need. There's a royal superiority to some Leos—you feel you deserve triple-ply cashmere, VIP all-access passes, and fifteen more minutes of fame than anyone else. Leos are the ultimate pretty prom princesses, party-givers, and party girls. If there's a game, sport, show, or party that's any good, chances are there is plenty of Leo energy making it happen. Just remember the little people who made it all possible.

Physical Domain: Leo rules the heart and mid-upper back. Back strain is a sign of stress, fever is a sign that you have to slow down and let the impurities burn out of your system. Although you're a fire sign, you can be heat-sensitive. Keep hydrated and take things slowly when you feel yourself begin to burn. If you're too busy showing off, partying, or pushing physical limits, you could strain your most vital muscle, your Leo heart.

What to Avoid in the Leo Workout: Looking at yourself instead of your fitness instructor.

Ideal Workout: You're in your element when you can be admired while you're keeping your heart strong and stretching your beautiful cat-like body. Pilates, for instance, is great for your back. You don't necessarily need an entourage but a few admirers and close friends make it all the more appealing. As long as there is a sense of fun and an inkling of VIP treatment, you'll be able to tolerate a little sweat and burn. Dancing highly charged salsa with a gorgeous guy is just about perfect.

Essential Workout Gear: Anything that makes you look hot.

Ultimate Trouble Spot: Upper back.

Workout Buddy Warning: You need optimistic, non-lazy friends who support your sunny side. As long as you're having fun, getting something done, and seeing results,

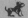

you're going to get along with anyone. You need to avoid dark and moody types because they cast a shadow over your sun. And you might be sensitive to other Leos who could steal your limelight!

If You Have a Personal Trainer:

1. Use a VIP, top-of-the line, celebrity-associated good-looker.

2. Praise is a must—forget the tough love type of trainer.

3. Use a guy you can flirt with and who clearly worships you.

Strategic Choices for Leo

The Leo Diet: Leos are not about food. Of course you need to eat well to fuel your fire (and for essentials like good skin, good looks, and party stamina). But you're not going to walk past every pizza place you see and wish you had a slice in your hand. Eating is either utilitarian (grab a yogurt before work so your stomach doesn't growl) or social (grab your friends for lunch so you won't be bored out of your mind). Leos enjoy the social interaction of entertaining and eating out. And this can be a shock to the pride of a Leo waistline.

As a fire sign, you have plenty of heat. You don't need spicy foods or stimulants but you might like them because it's all fuel to your flames. Watch for water weight gain associated with too much spice, or dehydration from too much coffee. You are sensitive to the water element since it is your nemesis.

Try not to let yourself get cold. You need to be warm or your energy will flag and you'll eat or drink to excess simply to keep warm. Opt for warm drinks like tea and not alcohol to fan your flames.

Since your heart is the center of your energy, you need to pay particular attention to healthy blood. Iron is your friend. Seek spinach and leafy greens, for sure, but the King of the Jungle is also a predator so if you crave red meat, it's okay to have the occasional moderate portion of steak or prime rib. Heart health is also maintained with a low-fat diet. Leos loathe butter substitutes and fat-free products though—imposters are not good enough for your royal blood. It's fine to eat the real thing—just keep those majestic portions under control.

zodiaction

1. **Warming spices.** Cinnamon, cayenne pepper, cumin. These will satisfy your love of spicy, flavorful foods with no negative side effects. Add cinnamon to your morning oatmeal or toast, cayenne pepper to your veggies and soups, and cumin to sauces and dressings.

2. **Organic rolled oats.** These are fiber-rich, and iron-stocked, and, first thing in the morning, they provide a steady fuel for your royal fires.

3. **Cooling vegetables.** Cucumbers, water chestnuts, celery. You love and can tolerate heat, but often you lose your edge when you become overheated. Instead of grabbing a cold soda or iced tea (both stimulants, which will only make you hotter in the long run), let cooling, water-based veggies keep you balanced.

Diet Vice: Fancy desserts.

Signature Spa Treatment: Hot stone massage.

Complementary Therapy: Alexander technique.

Mindfulness Mantra: When my heart is filled with light the world is filled with love.

Leo is the lifter of spirits. You are here to share your light and love, to set an example of bravery, resilience, and hope. The obligation of leadership can be tiring, especially when you feel down or stressed out. People will want to be near you just to get a little time in your sunshine. It's hard to keep up that light all the time, and when your energy flags it's time to retreat and let your flame revive. You don't need a long time because you're strong and lionhearted, but a good ruler knows when strategic retreat is the best choice. Don't let your vanity or your party-girl mission get in the way of taking care of yourself. Being overexposed is not good for your image, and letting people see you weak is simply unacceptable. Turn on that love light when you're feeling strong and able to share yourself. We love it when you do.

Leo in a Nutshell

MIND: You are a clear thinker and smart strategist when you're focused on a cause. You're also honest and kind, approachable, but dignified. Like many rulers, you don't always share what's on your mind but you remember what you need to know—kindnesses, bravery, integrity. You also do not forgive easily when people are rude, vulgar, or insulting. After all, the attitude and mind-set of royalty is lofty and compassionate but ultimately judgmental.

BODY: You love your body. Of all the signs, Leo is the least prone to self-deprecation and insecurity. Cat-like, soft, practical, and pleasurable, your body's your temple. Leos often have a "mane" of hair framing their regal faces, commanding stature (even if you're small, you seem tall). If you sense you're not looking as good as you could, you'll immediately shift your diet and exercise. You can't tolerate being less than your best.

SPIRIT: You are the sun, a beacon of life force and vitality. You light up hearts with your smile and fearlessly displace shadow.

Allow your fire to burn brightly and share warmth and light with the world. There is no shadow when you face your fears.

A Leo Workout Story

Julia is a quintessential Leo. She works long hours at a fast-paced advertising firm, then jets straight to the gym for back-to-back fitness classes. *Then* she showers, primps, and powders in the ladies' locker room, readying herself for a night on the town—perhaps prowling for cuties with her pack-mates. Julia's energy is non-stop and this is a typical day, seemingly thriving on minuscule amounts of R&R.

There's a lot to be commended here. Julia's high energy is great, her time management skills are superb, and her workouts exceed all expectation. The one trouble spot is her exhibitionism in the ladies' locker room. The girl doesn't see how uncomfortable her excessive nakedness makes other people. You see, Julia doesn't just walk to and from the shower nude, she puts on her makeup, stares dreamily at the reflection in the mirror, strikes up conversation with others, answers her cell phone . . . in the buff. Like many Leos, Julia is incredibly in love with her body, but enough is enough, Ms. Leo—be clad in undergarments at least! It's important to respect others by mastering the art of discretion.

THE LEO "LIONESS" WORKOUT

The Leo workout is one of the highest energy workouts of *Zodiaction,* because you've got the stamina, and the deepest desire to be the best. Add your devotion to your body and wow, there is nothing you can't do.

THREE WORKOUT GOALS FOR LEO

1. Heart strength. Keep your heart of gold from tarnishing with a strong cardiovascular component.

2. Total back health (strength, flexibility, and alignment). Posture is key to a powerful presence and your spine wants to move like a cat.

3. Serious toning. Being admired is always a good thing; you want the trouble spots (belly, buns, and thighs) to be purr-fect.

Leo, you are very aesthetic-result driven. This means that if a certain workout gives you those beautiful bodylines and sexy abs, that's motivation enough. You'll do it gladly, and you'll give it your all! While most of the other signs need a push every now and then, you don't. If anything, you may need someone to step on the brakes for you. All of your attributes point to a two-step workout: one measure of *"Pouncing" Power Yoga* followed by the not-to-be-trifled-with *Triple Whammy Toning.*

WORKOUT PRESCRIPTION

Leos are capable of working out every single day of the week, but if you do, you can*not* do the same thing every day. Aside from the aforementioned Leo workout, try to experience non-formal workouts—where you get exercise away from the gym, with friends. Leo girls are fun-lovers. Get into the sunshine and have a ball, or a skate, or a run, or a power walk. No slouching around in a dark old gym. Fresh air stokes your fire and gives you all the more opportunity to meet new people and bask in admiration. Rainy days and cold weather could keep you indoors—and that's where a great dance studio comes in. Try African dancing—it's so grounding as well as toning. Or ballet—great for core-strengthening and channeling your inner cat with pas de chats. Anywhere you find music, people, and fun is a place you can work out. Repetition, boredom, or arrogant instructors will suck the life out of you, though, so screen your gyms and change up your routines—and you'll be the sleekest cat in town.

BEST TIME TO WORK OUT: High noon.

STEP 1: Pouncing Power Yoga. Yes, "Pouncing," because you are a lion and you are playful. Yes, "Power," because you've got it and want more of it. And yes, "Yoga," because you will conquer three fitness worlds at once: stretch, strength, and cardio. The following exercises are to be performed in their proper sequence and at a fast pace, while maintaining proper form. Ideally, you will flow through all of the poses ten times for what in yoga is called "vinyasa," a yoga circuit. As you transition from Downward-Facing Dog back to the start of the series, leap forward into Forward Bend, giving you an extra-fun pounce—nine pounces total by the time you've finished Step 1.

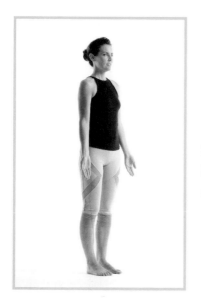

Mountain Pose

(PROVIDES A MOMENT OF CENTERING)

Stand tall with feet planted in parallel, palms of the hands facing forward. Hold for one breathing cycle (one inhale and one exhale).

Forward Bend

(RELEASES TENSION IN THE LOWER BACK)

Fold forward toward the floor. You may bend the knees if necessary. Hold for one breathing cycle (one inhale and one exhale).

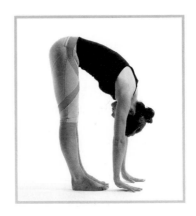

Plank

(TONES THE THIGHS, THE CORE, AND THE ARMS ALL AT ONCE)

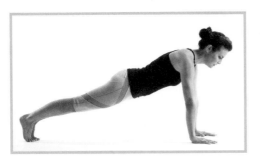

Plant both palms firmly and evenly on the floor, directly underneath the shoulders. Walk your feet back until your spine is parallel to the floor. Pull your abdominals in and squeeze your thigh muscles. Hold for one breathing cycle (one inhale and one exhale).

Warrior I

(TONES THE THIGHS, THE CORE, AND THE ARMS ALL AT ONCE)

Step your left foot forward into a sturdy lunge-like position, pivot your right heel inward. Smoothly, extend both arms joyously up overhead, elbows next to the ears. Hold for one breathing cycle (one inhale and one exhale).

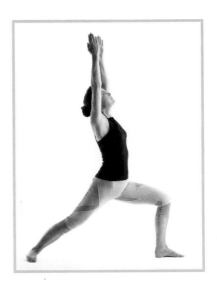

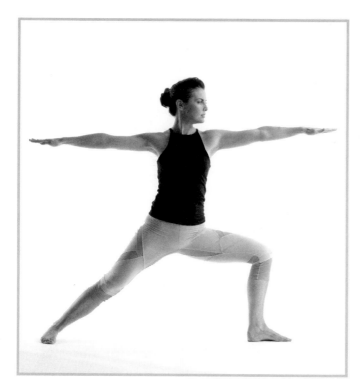

Warrior II

(TONES THE THIGHS, THE CORE, AND THE ARMS ALL AT ONCE)

Smoothly transition from Warrior I by keeping your lower body as is and turn your torso—opening up your upper body to the right. Arms are out at shoulder level. Hold for one breathing cycle (one inhale and one exhale).

Plank (again)

(TONES THE THIGHS, THE CORE, AND THE ARMS ALL AT ONCE)

Plant both palms firmly and evenly on the floor, directly underneath the shoulders. Walk your feet back until your spine is parallel to the floor. Pull your abdominals in and squeeze your thigh muscles. Hold for one breathing cycle (one inhale and one exhale).

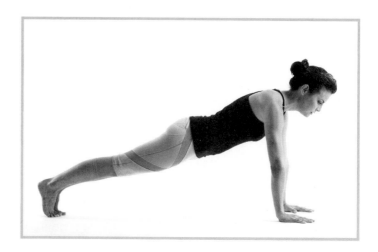

Chaturanga

(AN EXCELLENT UPPER BODY SCULPTOR)

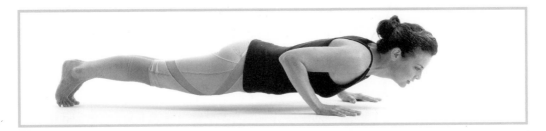

Simply lower the body toward the floor with complete control. Try to avoid dropping to the ground—the body should feel as though it is "surfing" above it. Your weight should be resting on the balls of your feet and the hands. Hold for one breathing cycle (one inhale and one exhale).

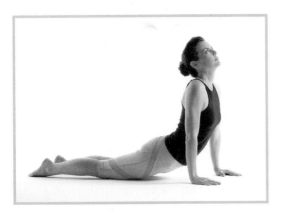

Upward-Facing Dog

(STRETCHES THE ENTIRE FRONT BODY)

Inhale and press the upper body up, toward the sky. Look up and press up, feel your front body open. Hold for one breathing cycle (one inhale and one exhale).

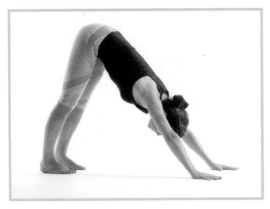

Downward-Facing Dog

(STRETCHES THE ENTIRE BACK BODY)

Exhale, hinge at the hips and lift the tailbone up toward the sky. The back, arms, and legs should all be straight. Hold for one breathing cycle (one inhale and one exhale). Remember to "pounce" into Forward Bend here, on your way back to Mountain Pose!

STEP 2: Triple Whammy Toning. Step 2 packs some serious muscular heat, just like Leo likes it. Do each of the three exercises until total fatigue sets in; you'll know it when you simply can't go on any longer. This may vary from day to day, so don't get hung up on a number; just feel your way through each exercise. Also, as in Step 1, these three exercises should be performed at a brisk pace. We're after running-for-the-train kind of urgency!

Knee Cross Crunch

(AN EXCELLENT EXERCISE FOR CORE STRENGTHENING)

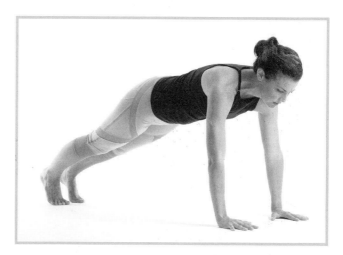

Begin in the Plank pose with your hands parallel to each other, palms directly underneath the shoulders. Engage your core muscles and squeeze your thigh muscles.

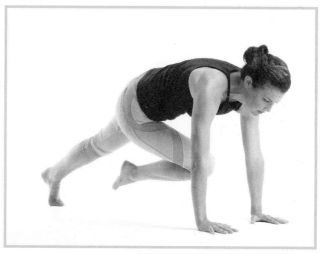

Exhale and bring your right knee toward your left shoulder. Quickly return the right leg down and exhale as you bring the left knee toward the right shoulder. Alternate right then left at a brisk pace, for a total of one hundred alternating crunches.

Butt Squeeze with Knee Flare

(LIFTS AND TONES THE BUTTOCK MUSCLES)

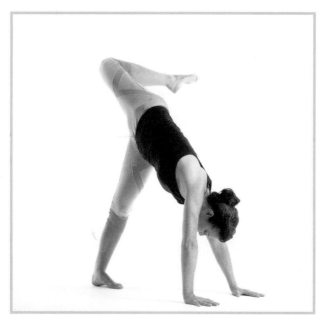

Find your Downward-Facing Dog position and raise your right leg up toward the ceiling. Flare your right hip open, bend your right knee, and try to reach your right foot toward your left butt cheek.

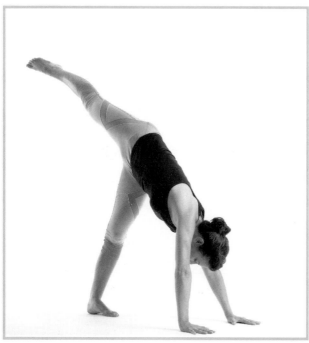

From this point, keeping the torso still, simply extend and then bend the right knee, strongly with a lot of vigor. Perform a series of twenty repetitions, then switch legs and be sure to repeat on the other side.

Double Leg Beat

(EFFECTIVELY TONES THE INNER THIGHS, LOWER BACK MUSCLES, AND BUTTOCKS)

Lie on your belly with legs extended straight behind you and hands underneath your chin. Relax your head, neck, and shoulders as much as possible throughout the exercise. Press your hips into the floor, lift both legs up off the floor and turn the heels slightly inward. Simply "click" your heels together, keeping both legs as straight as possible. Do one set of twenty repetitions and release.

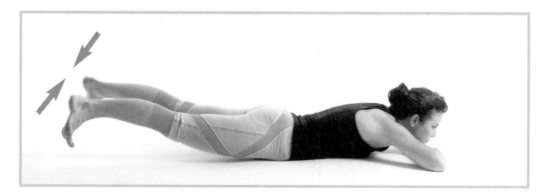

What's Ahead of Leo: A Star-Driven Five-Year Plan

2007 You're in the homestretch of a marathon inner transformation. It's been a challenging two years but this fall you're going to see it all pay off. While planets are winding down their pranks, take it easy. Keep your energy up with cardio but do not forget to find that inner peace. You'll want to be centered and strong when you receive your harvest.
Key Workout: Fat-burning Pilates and meditation.

2008 You're wildly healthy and robust this year. You'll need all that energy for the opportunities, shifts, and rewards ahead at work. Keep focused, be clear, and schedule well-balanced fun. Beware of overcrowding your social calendar, though. You need to stay on your game.
Key Workout: Tennis—you can work out and socialize at the same time.

2009   Your pretty head is going to turn a lot this year so keep that neck limber. So many admirers, so little time. Get lots of rest (use catnaps!) so you can keep up with high-pitched work and social demands. You might crave a mountain cabin, but you'll take the Vegas vacation instead. Party girl.
      Key Workout: Rock 'n' roll aerobics, cycling.

2010   It's a great year to make big changes, get big raises, and spend other people's money. Communications might seem a bit rocky so keep tabs on how well others react to your words. Leo determination and charisma can launch a whole business now. Ever thought of trying out for TV? Why not?
      Key Workout: Dancing for an audience or up on display.

2011   It's a good luck year but are you ready to gamble? Planets bring opportunities to travel and explore new areas of life. You have to straighten out those mini-conflicts before you go, though. It's a year to listen before you pass judgment. Kings try to be just but no one is right all the time. Hint, hint.
      Key Workout: Inner-focus and concentrated movement like ballet.

Signs of Life

Leo loves to be the life of the party. We all love you and your party-girl ways, but even you need to withdraw sometimes. Although you don't let many see your soft, vulnerable side, it's there. Read up on these signs to see how well they connect to the multifaceted you.

    Love life—Aquarius

    Career—Taurus

    Flirtation—Sagittarius

    Health—Capricorn

virgo-action

THE VIRGIN August 23—September 22

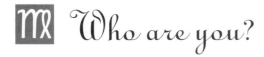 **Who are you?**

In One Word: KEEN

Symbol(s): The Virgin holding a handful of wheat, a symbol of the new harvest. Pure, efficient, discerning, Virgo is a Mercurial energy that solves problems, anticipates needs, and has extreme sensitivity. Small animals will steal your heart but stupid people will turn you cold.

Color: Harvest golds and yellows

Element: EARTH. As the second earth sign of the zodiac, you pick up from where Taurus left off. You provide earth energy to the world; what Taurus energy grew, your Virgo energy will reap. Your ability to sort out the wheat from the chaff is a gift: people, problems, clothing, food—if it exists, you can organize it. You have clear taste preferences; one might say you're the picky girl of the zodiac. Some Virgos are messy but all of you have an earth order in your own way. Food, diet, and exercise are especially important to you. When you're out of whack emotionally or intellectually, you will feel it physically.

Energy: MUTABLE. Earth in a mutable (changeable) form is what makes you so good at cutting through the world's BS. You are very sensitive to people and atmospheres. You're a bit of a psychic sponge, picking up others' vibes when they're in trouble.

zodiaction

When that happens it makes you super-stressed and means you're not giving enough time to yourself. You're the least grounded of the earth signs and when you've hit the wall Virgo meltdowns are legendary (it's the straw that breaks the Virgo's back). Poor digestion is a trusty clue that you're holding way too much stress inside. If you're erratic, you're not in control of your energy. Of course, the best solution for you is watching your diet and fitness. And that's what this is all about!

Psychic Domain: Virgo rules service, health, food, pets, servants, employees, and work. While Virgos can be one of the most serious signs, you're also the funniest—your fast mind produces a whip-cracking wit—hello Virgo Hugh Grant! You are tough on yourself though, because you see what could be made better. Virgo is ultimately a methodical perfectionist—and it's a job never done. The world desperately needs Virgos, with your quick eye, determination, and ability to fix tough problems. You're going to be overwhelmed by the needy, but to care for others you have to care for yourself too.

Physical Domain: Virgo rules the digestive tract and your energy rules assimilation. In practical terms, this means that you excel in taking in food, information, basic stuff, sorting it out, using what's good, and discarding what's not. If any sign was prone to Irritable Bowel Syndrome (IBS), constipation, colitis, or just random bouts of indigestion, it's you. When you're flowing well, your energy is unparalleled; your body is the most efficient machine on the planet. But when you're stressed, tired, or sick, you need to be very gentle on your digestive tract and let yourself rest back to normal.

What to Avoid in the Virgo Workout: Setting unrealistic goals and getting down on yourself for missing them. (And . . . long lines, overcrowded classes, smelly gyms, and dirty shower rooms—anything that adds stress!)

Ideal Workout: Totally efficient, full body conditioning with a concentration on abdominals. The Virgo workout should be a de-stressing and de-toxing experience. As a mutable sign, you're going to need a program with variety. The place for variation is in cardio, which is what you need to shake off all the thoughts and lists marching around your head. Repetitive cardio running, Elliptical training, biking, swimming, and other activities that lull you into a trance-like state help. Once you feel those endorphins going and you've got some "can-do" optimism, you can turn to body sculpting. That's where you find your center. Lucky for Virgo, one great workout is so powerful that it establishes a productive vibe in you for the remainder of the day.

Essential Workout Gear: Clean, good-looking, lean sweats with comfy shoes.

Ultimate Trouble Spot: Belly.

Workout Buddy Warning: You don't *need* a workout buddy but if you choose to include someone, he or she must keep up with you, and not just physically. You want your partner to match your mood, and your standards of cleanliness, agility, precision, and intelligence. You cannot under ANY circumstances work out with a complainer. You're better off on your own unless you're feeling relaxed and generous with your time—and when does that happen? It's fine to go to a gym with a friend, but try to work out independently without comparing how long you run, how much you lift, or how much you weigh.

If You Have a Personal Trainer:

1. Use someone with stunning credentials (i.e., years of experience and a long list of certifications). He or she needs to be knowledgeable about not just fitness, but *wellness* too.

2. Your trainer must be a little nitpicky, giving you specifics about how to hold a weight, how to breathe, perfect alignment, etc. These kinds of acute details will bore other signs, but they secretly fill Virgos with glee.

3. Any trainer must be clean (absolutely no dirt underneath his or her nails), smell good, and not get into your personal space.

Strategic Choices for Virgo

The Virgo Diet: So totally important. If there's anyone who lives up to the concept of "You are what you eat," it's you. But make no mistake—Virgos are not saints. Taco Bell, fast food burgers, even super-frosted donuts can pass through the lips of the most food-conscious Virgos. As the pickiest eaters of the zodiac, you have your diehard favorite foods. Chicken-fried steak? Boston cream pie? Whatever it is, you're not about to give up something you love. The thing about Virgo is that you feel every atomic inch of what you eat. Your digestive system will wince at foods that are too rich, too fatty, or too heavy. You're sensitive and you know it.

But all is not lost. You can still indulge on little binges if you're in good shape. If you keep your diet mainly on track, any little diversion in indulgence will be tolerated without too much pain. If you do give in to cravings or go on a serious binge, however, you will find that your waistline responds quickly with added inches and your regularity goes right into the trash.

You can keep yourself on track and happy with a lot of fiber. Whole grains, seeds, and some nutty breads (you rule wheat, after all) can help. If you happen to be sensitive to wheat (gluten is not every Virgo's friend) find a grain that works for you. Chew well—your digestion starts in your mouth.

Meats are not ideal for Virgos. Red meat in particular is very taxing on your digestive system. However, there is no use ignoring a craving for a good burger when you really need it. Just don't make it a dietary staple. If you do want to eat meat (chicken, pork, game, or beef) make sure it is prepared well and try to make the surrounding meals vegetarian.

Virgos need clean restaurants and conscious cooks. Carry food that you prepare with you so that you don't have to rely on others' standards for hygiene. You are the sign most prone to food-poisoning, so be careful what you order and how it's cooked. Go ahead; ask the waiter anything and everything. He's been waiting for a Virgo to test his knowledge.

Here is one more vital piece of dietary advice. Food is digested more efficiently at body temperature, therefore cold fluid can slow down your digestive process. If you must drink while eating, make it room temperature water and skip the ice.

THE TOP THREE ITEMS TO SHOP FOR:

1. **Flaxseed (to sprinkle on salads and top off your cereals).** Flaxseed is high in fiber and adds a tasty crunch.

2. **Root vegetables like yams, potatoes, carrots, and beets.** High in fiber and easily digested, root veggies are all-star forms of fuel. Be sure to prepare them as simply as possible, with limited salt, butter, and cheese.

3. **Ginger tea (aids digestion) and chamomile tea (soothes the stomach lining).** These are great teas to ingest before bed, especially if your dinner was a five-course meal.

Diet Vice: Hot dog from a street vendor.

Signature Spa Treatment: Shiatsu massage.

Complementary Therapy: Colonic irrigation or a vegetable juice fast.

Mindfulness Mantra: I can give to others best when I have given enough to myself.

Virgo is the energy of purpose and accomplishment. You find a sense of purpose every day just waking up. When you're "on," Ms. Perfectionist, you're the best employee around, the greatest critic, the most compassionate friend—you name it, you're the best. When you're "off," though, your perfectionist tendencies will work against you. You're down on yourself, you're crabby, and you can lash out at anyone who might ask you for the time. That's because you tend to take on too much—and when you do that you go on auto-shutdown. You can't solve the world's problems although, frankly, you are smart enough to figure them all out. What you need is moderation, to take your life one step at a time, to be selective about those you help, and not to expect immediate gratification when you make an effort. You're also prone to distraction. Your superhero gift of intuition sends off an alarm every time a needy human or animal comes onto your radar. Turn off that intuition once in a while.

Virgo in a Nutshell

MIND: Smart, snappy, witty, sharp, keen, penetrating. You have exactly what it takes to analyze and size up any problem or situation. Within five seconds, you know that infomercial product is a hoax. Your mind is a gift to us all—you can cut through any amount of jibber-jabber doubletalk and nail down a problem. (Why aren't there more of you in Congress?!) Your mind is your friend until you turn it against yourself. One minute you'll talk yourself into a nice little snack and right after you eat it your mind is telling you that you made a mistake. Turn off that mind once in a while so it can reset.

BODY: Your body is your temple and you need to show it respect. The minute you slack off on diet, fitness, or rest you will find yourself in a sorry state of anxiety. You're sensitive to the slightest imbalance like too many French fries or not enough water.

zodiaction

A Virgo Workout Story

Meet Helena. She's 5'10", worked as a runway model back in the 1970s, and is now the proud mother of two teenagers. Helena has never been overweight. In fact, she had to work extra hard to put on the appropriate amount of weight during each of her pregnancies. She walks every day to and from work and gladly pays the extra cost for organic foods. If you ask her if she's been content with her body, she'll say yes, except for one spot—her waistline. It's driven her mad over the years. She's tried everything, billions of crunches, special diets, liver cleanses, and fasts. Nothing seems to flatten her belly for good.

Enter Pilates. Yes, Pilates has been hailed as the ultimate in abs. Its secret for success is simple. It pulls muscles in (not out), uses the breath (for added energy), and sculpts the core muscles evenly (the abs *and* lower back together). In addition to that, Pilates epitomizes the "less is more" philosophy.

Remember the billions of crunches? Well, Helena bid them a big adieu—she's seen the light. Just several Pilates exercises each day has gotten the job done. Now, in her mid-forties, Helena has her all-time most rockin' bod.

THE VIRGO "PERFECT SYNERGY" WORKOUT

Every workout in *Zodiaction* is a complete workout. Virgo's is no exception, but at first glance you may believe otherwise. You see, Virgo's workout is a complete total body routine but *appears* to be exclusively about abs. This is intentional. We know the ultimate motivator (and the ultimate trouble spot) for Ms. Goddess of the Harvest is your belly, and we use this bit of info to attract and maintain your attention. If you have a strong core, your power center is thus strong, making your emotional or intellectual energy harmonious. (Plus, those abs look exquisite!)

We've broken the Virgo workout into three sections, to be done in sequential order. First up, a *Detoxifying Power Walk*. This can be done outdoors or indoors and should without a doubt be brisk. We need you to break a sweat to release those toxins. The second step is an *Abdominal with Weights* routine. Of course this will blast your abs into incredible shape, but it will also provide great resistance training for your upper body. And the third component is *Stretching for Improved Digestion*. These four stretches help the kidneys, liver, stomach, and intestines thrive, so your digestion thrives.

WORKOUT PRESCRIPTION

Virgo girls want effective, efficient workouts that provide real results. Workouts can be goal-oriented as long you don't set them unrealistically or obsessively. If anything, Virgo is the compulsive energy of the zodiac and you should be careful not to get too crazy about hitting the gym. If you've got a fever, stay home. If you're overtired, don't push yourself. It's not many signs where we have to tell people to take it easy, but you want to be sure not to get too nuts about getting in your reps or taking off that last half a pound. If you turn that "must-do" energy inside out, you'll be the biggest slacker in the universe (of course it won't last, but who needs to go there at all?). Go easy on yourself; give yourself time to work out, set goals with enough gray area that you won't get sulky if you miss them. You have all it takes to stay in great shape your whole life. So go for it—with an easy attitude. Do you have to work out every day? No. Should you? No. We believe four or five days per week is ideal for you.

BEST TIME TO WORK OUT: First thing.

STEP 1: Detoxifying Power Walk. Aim for forty-five minutes, go brisk (pump those arms!), and wear an extra layer of clothing, so you heat things up. We recommend that you sweat. You're not a fan of sweating excessively, but you do deeply desire a toxin-free body. Let your desire for cleanliness lure you down the road.

STEP 2: Abs with Weights. Yes, the focus is on your core with an added bonus in upper body toning at the same time. We recommend using a pair of 2–5 lb weights. Do the recommended exact amount of reps too; no more, no less.

Basic Crunch

(EFFECTIVELY TONES THE ABDOMINALS)

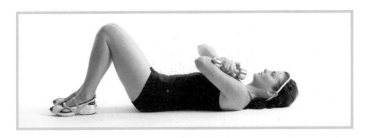

Lie on your back with your feet planted in parallel, knees bent, and head resting comfortably on the floor. With one weight in each hand, crisscross your forearms on your upper chest.

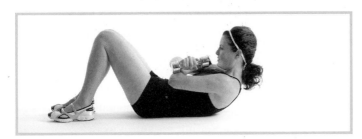

Exhale and curl the head and shoulders off the floor by squeezing your abdominal muscles in toward the spine. Inhale and return to the starting position. Repeat ten times.

The Teaser

(EFFECTIVELY TONES THE ABDOMINALS)

Sit upright with your feet planted in parallel and your arms extended out in front of you.

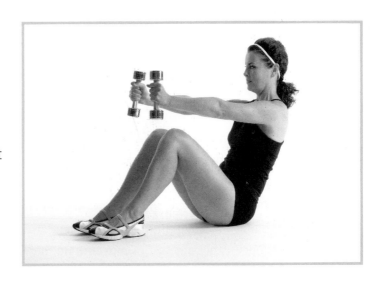

Exhale and curl your spine down to the floor slowly. Inhale and raise the arms up overhead. Exhale and return to the starting position by curling your spine up toward the ceiling. For the duration of this movement, the feet, knees, and legs stay still. Repeat ten times.

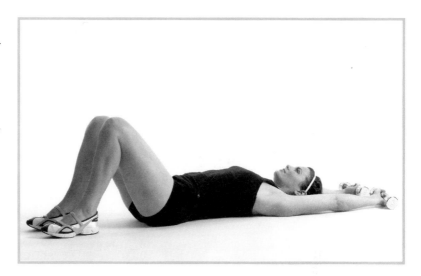

The Canoe

(STRENGTHENS THE ENTIRE CORE)

Start in a seated upright position with your feet planted in parallel. Grasp both weights with both hands and lean back, as if in a bucket seat. Exhale and twist the torso to the

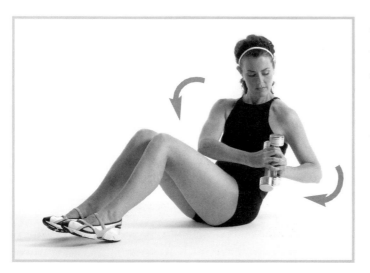

right, then smoothly transition to the left by twisting in the other direction. The movement is very similar to rowing in a canoe. Repeat twenty times alternating, for ten repetitions on each side.

The Boxer

(TONES THE CORE AND THE UPPER ARMS SIMULTANEOUSLY)

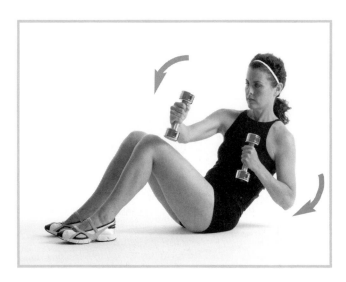

Begin seated with one weight in each hand. Plant your feet in parallel, with both knees comfortably bent. Lean back as if in a bucket seat. Exhale and punch the right arm across the body toward the left, then exhale and punch the left arm across the body toward the right, twisting the torso as you go. Alternate side to side for a total of twenty repetitions, ten on each side.

The Scoop Hold

(TONES THE CORE AND PROVIDES A BALANCE)

Balance on your hips by picking up your feet and slightly scooping the belly. Hold both weights with both hands and straighten them as much as possible overhead. The more "up" you go, the more challenging, so you be the judge; you can customize your level of intensity. Hold for sixty seconds and then release. (You always have the option of performing the exercise without the hand weights.)

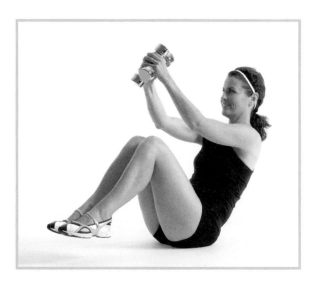

STEP 3: Stretching for Improved Digestion.

Seated Spine Twist

(EXCELLENT STRETCH FOR FLUSHING THE KIDNEYS WITH FRESH OXYGEN WHILE AT THE SAME TIME STRETCHING OUTER THIGH, LOWER BACK, AND NECK MUSCLES)

Sit upright with spine tall and extended. Bend your left knee underneath you on the floor and cross the right leg on top. Try to plant the right foot near the left knee. Then simply twist the torso toward the right. Look over your right shoulder and hold for sixty seconds. Release, then switch sides. Be sure to change the legs as well as the direction of the twist.

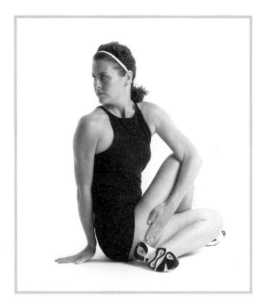

Single Leg Tortoise Pose

(MASSAGES THE ASCENDING AND DESCENDING COLON AS YOU STRETCH LOWER BACK AND GLUTES)

Start by bringing your left leg forward into a kneeling position. Extend the right leg long behind you. Slowly begin to drape your upper body over your front leg, using

your arms for control. Once you arrive at your deepest stretch, hold for sixty seconds. Gracefully roll your back up and switch legs. Repeat the entire process once more with the right leg forward.

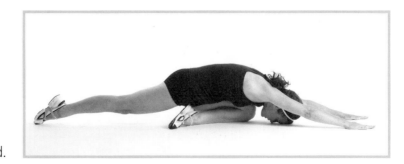

Happy Baby Pose (Ananda Balasana)

(MASSAGES THE LIVER WHILE STRETCHING THE HAMSTRINGS)

Lie on your back with your head and shoulders comfortably resting on the floor. Bring both knees in toward the chest. Grab hold of your feet. Flex both feet and apply a bit of pressure, subtly forcing the knees down. Hold for sixty seconds and release.

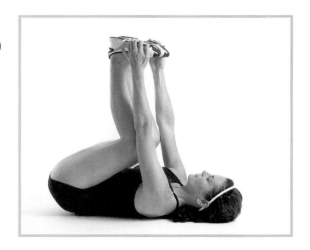

Seated "Hoola"

(RIDS THE CORE OF TENSION AND INCREASES CIRCULATION TO THE ABDOMEN)

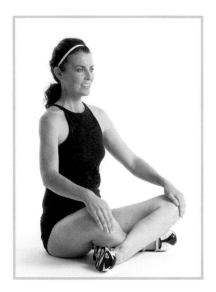

Begin by sitting in a cross-legged position with your hands delicately resting upon your knees.

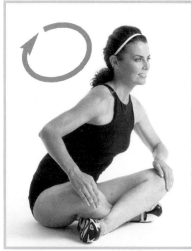

Without lifting your hips off the floor, "roll" your torso in a clockwise circle. Repeat five times, then reverse the direction and go counterclockwise for another five repetitions.

What's Ahead of Virgo: A Star-Driven Five-Year Plan

2007   You're a bit of a homebody and a little shy of crowds as the planets push you into reevaluating your life. Your key to happiness is rest and rejuvenating activities. Steer clear of rigid rules and relentless whiners.
Key Workout: Jumping rope in your backyard, long bike rides in the countryside.

2008   Part of you wants to party like a rock star and another voice in you is saying stick to the ashram. If you can balance wild flirtations, risk-taking sports, and late hours with a healthy diet and frequent intervals of rest, you'll be just fine. But who are we kidding?
Key Workout: If it's fun, you'll do it. Crank up the tunes and dance around your living room.

2009   Saturn starts to finish with your sign. If you think you were seriously intense before, you're even more so now. Do. Not. Be. So. Hard. On. Yourself. You're so smart, capable, and loving, and it's critical to remember that. No one puts pressure on you like you do yourself. So cut it out.
Key Workout: Anything without rules—like a leisurely hike or bike ride.

2010   After all the work you've done on yourself, you finally get what you deserve. No, it's not a stress test—it's love, happiness, and peace. Planets offer you some time off from Herculean tasks, but you're never one to turn down a challenge. Try to remember that there's no guilt in being content.
Key Workout: Power walking outside.

2011   Money matters and big jobs come up this year, and planets make you open to new opportunities with better paychecks. Nothing comes easily, though, so it's a great time to balance stress and ambition with detachment and patience. Working out is key.
Key Workout: A mind–body-type workout like yoga or Qigong with an inspiring instructor.

zodiaction

Signs of Life

Virgo, you no doubt get tired of being told how efficient and exacting you are. We love your wit too, but you know there's more to you than that. Let yourself explore more dimensions by reading the signs that rule the many layers of your life. You've got a lot going on in there!

Love life—Pisces

Career—Gemini

Flirtation—Capricorn

Health—Aquarius

libra-action

THE BALANCE September 23–October 22

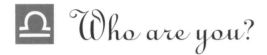 *Who are you?*

In One Word: HARMONIOUS

Symbol(s): Blind justice, holding scales. Libra is the sign of peace, partnership, and balance. It searches for the other side of the story before weighing the truth. Of course, the two sides tend to struggle to win over the other, the perpetual "well, on one hand . . . and then on the other hand . . ." That's why making choices and decisions is Libra's dilemma.

Color: Watermelon-rind green

Element: AIR. As the second of the three air signs, you prefer concepts and ideas to the Gemini's love of mundane facts. You have a very smart, capable mind that easily grasps complicated thoughts and delves into details. Libra is the sign of the law, and many Libras make great lawyers. Your capacity to right wrongs and embrace justice gives an edge in argument over any other sign—if only the thought of conflict didn't make you want to fly away. Like other air signs, Libra has a problem staying grounded. You live in your head and float into the theoretical when you need to be focused on a real-world problem. It must be all that conflict avoidance. Libras are totally charming, though, and your considerable smarts make you great friends and awesome mates.

zodiaction

Energy: CARDINAL. You're the third of four cardinal energies of the zodiac and you exercise your sharpshooter aim in the element of air. If you have an idea, you give it full consideration before you share it with anyone. If you have a problem, you think it through and solve it. You're the most successful strategic thinker of the zodiac because you apply your ability to understand both sides of an argument, weigh the information, and express a strong case for the Right Answer. Of course, that is when you can actually make up your mind. The toughest scenario for a Libra is to need resolution but be unable to find it. Often just choosing what you'll eat for dinner can be debilitating. Libra's challenge, as a cardinal air sign, is to settle on an answer, even if you're not absolutely sure that you're right.

Psychic Domain: Libra girls are peace-loving, harmonious creatures who worship the holy trinity of hair, makeup, and fashion. Like Taurus, your planetary ruler is Venus, but instead of being about earthly delights, Libra is about thinking beautiful thoughts, promoting justice, and keeping the world as serene as possible while looking perfectly lovely. You can't stand disharmony or ugliness, and you'll avoid confrontation at almost any cost. You're a natural diplomat. When you're forced to fight, however, you almost always win. When you get to the point where you just can't take disequilibrium or conflict for one more second, you act to resolve it as swiftly and brutally as any five-star general. Then you go right back to being pretty, peace-loving you.

Physical Domain: Libra rules the kidneys and lower back—it's all about balance! Since the universe has a dry sense of humor, you will notice that fellow Libra girls usually have some problems with grace. They fall off high heels, they trip up stairs, and they fall over in yoga classes—physical balance is hard to strike. You can be sure that the more stressed you are, the klutzier you'll feel. Lower back problems are common to Libra stress. Massage is effective, but meditating is even better. Inner peace brings serenity to your life *and* your limbs.

What to Avoid in the Libra Workout: Intramural rugby, boxing gyms, and Venice Beach, California (and any other places of grit, crowds, and rough-edged muscle).

Ideal Workout: Stretch and balance work with low-impact cardio to quiet your mind and strengthen your focus on inner balance and serenity. Pilates work is great for Libras since it really focuses on your core issues. While ballet classes in the strictest sense might be too stressful, ballet-type stretches will improve your posture and your balance. Ballet will also provide excellent range of motion for your hips, which will help balance out your lower body. Libra girls don't like to look unkempt, so low-impact (easy on the back) walking or cross-training is a great way to keep trim and blow off some steam.

Essential Workout Gear: Designer anything that makes you look pretty.

Ultimate Trouble Spot: Lower back tightness and lack of range of motion.

Workout Buddy Warning: Libra rules partnership, thus a workout with company is desirable . . . unless your buddy is argumentative, sloppy, or stupid. You will only add stress to your life if you don't respect your workout mate. You also like group exercise classes, which could be an alternative for you to get social with people while you sweat.

If You Have a Personal Trainer:

1. You need compliments, and plenty of them.

2. Your trainer must understand lower backs and how to strengthen and protect them.

3. Preferably you'll have a cute trainer but not cuter than you.

Strategic Choices for Libra

The Libra Diet: Libra girls are prone to vanity and therefore you're not one of the signs that tend toward overeating. Even though food isn't your thing, you're close enough to the sign of Virgo that you could be a picky eater. Libra girls like their comfort food, like macaroni and cheese, mashed potatoes, and hot rolls with butter—who doesn't? But Libras are air signs and cannot afford to get weighed down by heavy dough and sludgy carbs. You don't want all your energy in your stomach weighing you down when you want to think clearly.

Being an air sign, you also possess a bit of a sweet tooth. Moderation is the key to your good looks and trim figure. But if you're stressed out, sugar is your therapy: lollipops, Jolly Ranchers, and any other hard candies that take a while to finish are your best friends.

Now, here comes our spiel about kidneys. Yup, kidneys. Libra rules these organs, located in your lower back region, that cleanse blood and rid the body of impurities. Healthy liquids like water, cranberry juice, and teas—and lots of them—will help keep Libra's kidneys in tip-top shape, which in turn means: Your skin? Clear and gorgeous. Your energy? *Up and at 'em.* Your spirit? Focused and balanced. Water-dense fruits like watermelon and grapefruit make great Libra snacks. Basically, whatever is going on in your kidneys is going to show up in the rest of your body/mind/spirit, and FAST. Be aware of this and eat accordingly.

There is one obvious substance that taxes your kidneys, Libra, and that is alcohol. Since Libra rules distillation (i.e., wine and spirits), we've got a distinct dilemma when it comes to you and booze. You enjoy those cocktails, especially in social circumstances, but balance and moderation are necessary when it comes to ingesting cocktails of any kind. We don't need you to swear off drinking—you're not "allergic" to Grey Goose—you're just sensitive to vodka, gin, whiskey, and their cousins. Your kidneys are unequipped to handle large amounts of alcohol. Thus we recommend that you get into the habit of diluting all alcoholic beverages. Enjoy a wine spritzer instead of straight wine, put ice in your pint of beer, and when opting for a trendy cocktail tell the bartender to "go easy on the liquor" (remember, your glowing skin is at stake).

The vital piece of information to retain from this section is this: Libra's wellness is a direct result of her kidneys' wellness, and diet plays a monumental role in kidney wellness. You're very clued in to your balance, so use that insight when it comes to eating and drinking.

THE TOP THREE ITEMS TO SHOP FOR:

1. **Fresh parsley (note: not parsley flakes or dried parsley "herbs").** Parsley is a wonder food for kidney cleansing and it goes with just about anything. Put it on your pasta, in your soup and salad, on your baked halibut.

2. **Fresh lemons (note: not lemon juice or lemonade).** Much like fresh parsley, lemons are great for aiding kidney function. They add zing to just about everything. Great in salad dressings and squeezed over fish. Use a slice of lemon in your water and in your tea instead of sugar and milk.

3. **Fresh fish, like halibut, trout, sea bass, and tuna.** Go to a fish market if possible,

and avoid buying it at Shop 'n Save. You want the absolute best quality and the freshest catch. Fish is your best bet for animal-based protein. Get into the habit of *not* eating red meat, chicken, or pork, which can be abusive to Libra's kidneys. Also, try to avoid other seafood, like shrimp, king crab, and scallops. They sometimes have high levels of mercury, which may overburden your . . . you guessed it . . . your kidneys.

Diet Vice: Comfort food—fries, mac & cheese, eggs and bacon.
Signature Spa Treatment: Thai yoga massage is great for nurturing your lower back.
Complementary Therapy: Full day of beauty at a spa.
Mindfulness Mantra: The world is in harmony when I am serene.

Libra is all about beauty, peace, harmony, and aesthetic appreciation. Libra girls love art, music, and most especially love. The sad fact that the world is a place of conflict, noise, and imperfection can stress out an otherwise happy Libra. Libras cannot understand why anyone would voluntarily be disagreeable. Why would anyone want to fight? Certainly you wouldn't unless forced to. It is a bewildering fact that life has unpleasantness in it, and you'll go to great lengths to avoid it, but no matter how smart and skillful you are, not everything is beautiful. The only place that harbors true, constant beauty within your complete control is inside you. Rather than seek beauty outside of yourself, or through cosmetics, clothing, shoes, hair, or jewelry, you need to find your center. That sacred space inside your heart contains all the beauty, peace, and harmony you crave.

Libra in a Nutshell

MIND: Intelligent, embracing, skillful, and strategic, your mind is your best friend. Your natural impulse for balance can cause you to mull too much, thinking through problems with what-ifs until you've forgotten why you care. When your brain goes on overload, drop the energy down to your heart. Your heart can tell you anything from what to order in a restaurant to big decisions like if you want to marry your boyfriend—but you have to stop thinking to hear the answer.

BODY: You know you're cute. Libra girls take care of their looks and take pride in their appearance. That isn't to say you have the healthiest habits in the zodiac, though. Be careful not to rely too heavily on cosmetics to cover sleep deprivation or bad eating habits. Your natural good looks are really your best option.

SPIRIT: You see the beauty in the world and smooth over the problems with careful thought. Resolving conflict is the key to inner balance.

Share your vision of beauty with the world.
Allow for differences, take action for justice and you will find the peace you crave.

A Libra Workout Story

Last year, Jennifer registered for the fifth annual *Save Tibet 5K Run/Walk.* It's "nothing serious," her Aries friend confided, elaborating that last year, the fundraiser included mothers running while pushing strollers and complete novices wearing their iPods (a very amateur thing to do, apparently). "There are lots of walkers," she was told. "And anyway, it's just a 5K." So Jennifer, leery at first, was convinced. She's never been into running for sport, but hey, it'll be fun and social, plus people are joining forces for justice—all very motivating for Ms. Libra.

Flash forward to race day. Jennifer shows up with her four friends and a full face of makeup. Lip gloss in pocket. There are colorful banners everywhere and a live band playing "Beautiful Day" by U2. *It is a beautiful day,* she thinks to herself.

As the runners make their way to the starting line, Jennifer and her four compadres huddle together, all giddy with pre-race butterflies. A few announcements are made by the race committee and then the gun goes off. As Jennifer's four buddies sprint fast to secure a space at the front of the pack, she is left in the dust.

The race might not have been competitive by an Aries standard, but to a Libra, it might as well be the Olympics. So much for hanging with friends.

THE LIBRA "HARMONY" WORKOUT

Libra girls don't want to work out as much as "work on" the body. So rather than a punishing, grueling challenge, you need to respectfully tone and strengthen. Everything must be presented in a peaceful manner, thus the title *Harmony Workout*. For Libra, there is no room for rushing around or a panicky attitude.

The *Harmony Workout* should take about thirty minutes—a perfect fit for Libra—since that's all you need and all you are motivated for. Do the three parts in the presented sequence for the most harmonious results.

THREE WORKOUT GOALS FOR LIBRA

1. Achieve overall energetic balancing.

2. Improve lower back strength and stretch.

3. Stretch on the physio-ball (a better balance bonus!).

WORKOUT PRESCRIPTION

Libra girls would rather live in the past, when standing on a machine with a vibrating belt would trim the waist. Hard work, sweat, and intense training sessions are not a strong enticement to get you to the gym. But here's the good news: you can still stay fit and trim in your own beauty-driven world, walking in the park while listening to soothing music, or watching a gripping movie from the treadmill.

Stay motivated and keep to your workout plan in the way you would put a dress on layaway. Do a little bit every day and soon you'll reach your goals. And you'll look great in whatever dress you do decide to wear.

BEST TIME OF DAY TO WORK OUT: Midday—balancing morning and afternoon energy.

STEP 1: Ten minutes of Jumping Rope. Feel the rhythm and get into a smooth groove. If you are *sans* rope, try "air" jumping. Simply pretend you are jumping an invisible rope. Be light on your toes and avoid making loud thudding noises with your feet. You can do this by slightly engaging your abdominals (imagine you are wearing a corset). Jumping rope is an excellent way to get into a fat-burning zone (and break a sweat!), quickly and easily. To keep yourself honest, set the alarm on your mobile phone to sound in exactly ten minutes.

STEP 2: Pilates for a Beautiful Back. The following five exercises should be performed in a fluid motion. No jerky movements allowed! And as with all Pilates exercise, breathing is central, so be sure to pay extra attention to the inhale/exhale cues. Be in the moment as you perform these exercises, to make them feel extra peaceful.

Open Leg Rocker

(THIS EXERCISE RELAXES THE NERVE ENDINGS OF THE SPINE, WHILE FLATTENING THE ABDOMINALS AND IMPROVING BALANCE)

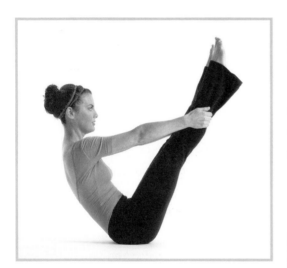

Sit down, bend your knees in toward the body, and gently grab hold of your ankles. Now lift your feet off the floor and balance on your hips. Once you've established your equilibrium, extend both legs straight, hip-distance apart.

Inhale and gracefully roll onto your back, all the way to your shoulder blades. Exhale and roll back up to your balance point. Try to avoid tapping your feet against the floor. Repeat eight times total.

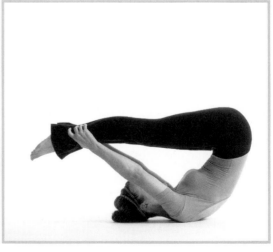

Roll Over

*(THIS EXERCISE DEEPLY STRETCHES
AND STRENGTHENS THE LOWER BACK MUSCLES)*

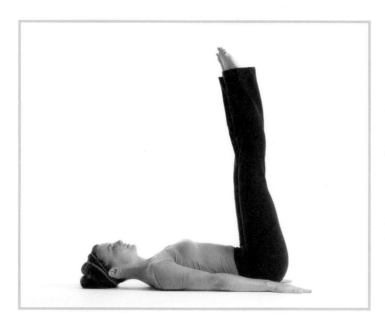

Lie on your back with your arms along your sides on the floor and your legs extended straight up toward the ceiling. Point your toes and completely relax your head and neck.

Exhale and lift your hips up, bringing your legs up and over your head, parallel to the floor. Inhale and hold, then exhale and slowly roll the spine back to the starting position. Inhale and pause at the starting position. Repeat eight times total.

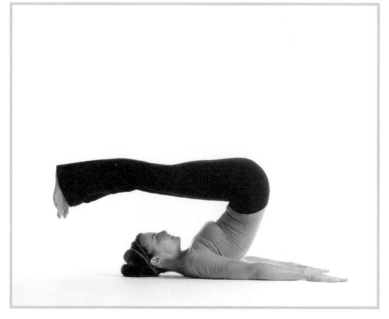

Side Scoop

(THIS EXERCISE STRETCHES AND STRENGTHENS THE HARD-TO-REACH
SIDE BACK MUSCLES, AND PROVIDES A GREAT CRUNCH FOR THE OBLIQUES)

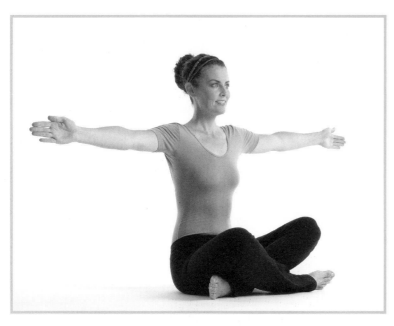

Begin in the cross-legged position with the spine upright and arms extended out, like airplane wings. Keep the hips "glued" to the floor for the duration of the exercise.

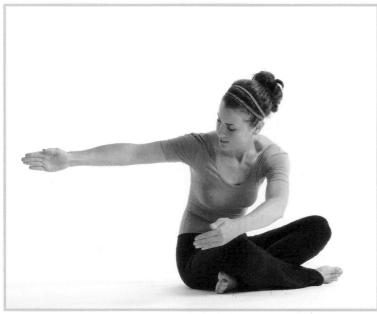

Exhale and "scoop" the belly as you reach the left arm across the body toward the floor underneath the right shoulder. Inhale and return to the starting position. Then exhale, scoop the belly, and reach the right arm across the body toward the floor underneath the left shoulder. Inhale and return to the starting position. Alternate for a total of ten repetitions.

Side-Lying Twist (from Side Plank position)

(A GREAT STRENGTHENER OF THE ENTIRE CORE)

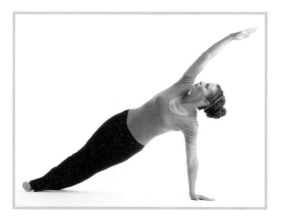

Position the body in a Side Plank pose by balancing on the left arm and the left outer edge of the foot. The abdominals must be engaged at all times. Reach the right arm up overhead, and then place the right foot slightly in front of the left, to assist with balance.

Keep your lower body still and exhale the torso forward, reaching the right arm up and over an imaginary beach ball. Inhale and return to the starting position. Do a set of eight, then switch sides and perform a second set on the other side.

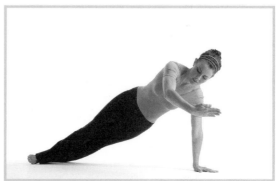

Swimming

(THIS EXERCISE PROMOTES SYMMETRY BETWEEN THE UPPER, MIDDLE, AND LOWER BACK MUSCLES)

Lie on your belly with legs and arms extended. Lift all four limbs off the floor to begin. Now kick the left leg and right arm up toward the ceiling. Immediately switch and kick the right leg and the left arm up toward the ceiling. Alternate for a total of twenty repetitions, ten on each side.

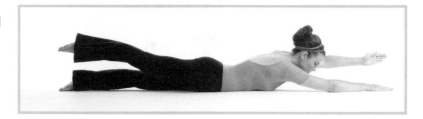

zodiaction

STEP 3: Stretching with a Physio-Ball. The physio-ball might as well have been invented by a Libra for Libras. It's got Libra written all over it. No matter what you do with the physio-ball, you're playing with your equilibrium, fine-tuning it every moment. While the following five stretches are passive, keeping your balance is active. A perfect balance.

Back Bend

(PROVIDES A SAFE AND SUBTLE BACK BEND)

Start by sitting on the ball with both feet firmly planted on the ground. Slowly begin to drape your back over the ball by leaning back. Stretch your arms back toward the floor. Hold the stretch for sixty seconds.

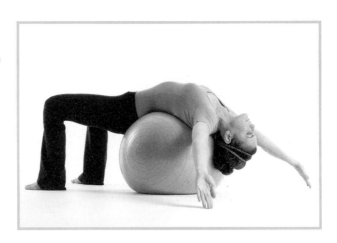

Chest Stretch

(STRETCHES THE MUSCLES OF THE CHEST)

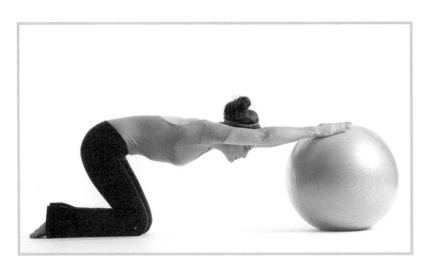

Kneel next to the ball and place the palms of your hands on top of it. Keeping your elbows straight, roll the ball away from you until your back is parallel to the floor. Hold the stretch for sixty seconds.

Seated Twist

*(THE SEATED TWIST IS A NICE WAY TO STRETCH THE CORE MUSCLES
AND RELEASE TENSION FROM THE LOWER BACK AND NECK)*

Sit atop the ball and cross your right leg over your left knee. Keep your spine straight and find your balance. Now twist the torso toward the right, grab the right knee with your left hand, and look over your right shoulder. Hold for sixty seconds, then switch sides and repeat.

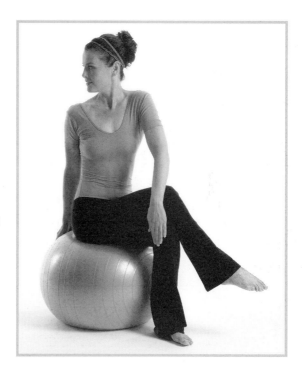

Accordion Stretch

*(STRETCHES THE LOWER BACK,
TONES THE ABDOMINALS)*

Place both palms firmly on the floor and kneel on the ball. Bring the chest in toward the knees and bring the hips down to the heels. You should feel your abdominals engage as your lower back muscles stretch. Hold for sixty seconds.

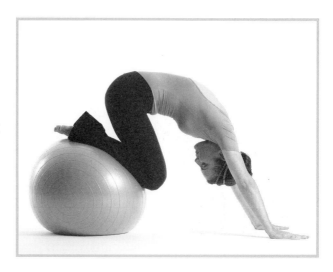

Side Stretch

[STRETCHES THE ENTIRE SIDE TORSO]

Kneel on the floor adjacent to the ball and allow your torso to drape over it. Be sure to keep your hips and shoulders in line with each other. Hold for sixty seconds and then switch sides and repeat.

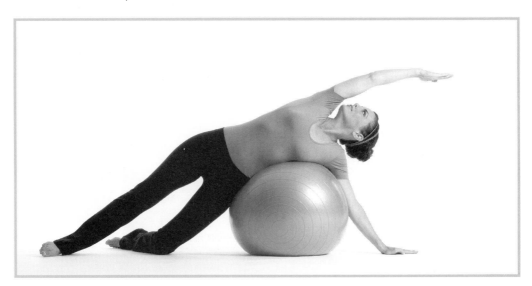

What's Ahead of Libra: A Star-Driven Five-Year Plan

2007   It's a year of constant ideas, parties, and achieving some big heartfelt goals. The long slog of challenge is behind you and you're ready to fall back onto a little carefree fun. Use your buoyant spirits to push your fitness program further.

   Key Workout: Group runs—maybe a 10K or even a mini-marathon.

2008   The atmosphere shifts to a homey need for private time. You just don't have the party stamina you used to and, to be quite honest, you don't like to be around many people. Enjoying time by yourself should wear a rut from your

couch to the kitchen, so take your solitude on the road and walk your dog—
or your boyfriend.

Key Workout: Long ambles in new territory.

2009 It's a tug-of-war with planetary powers of flirtation versus pulling the covers
over your head. Balance is tricky this year but here's the key: party hard, rest
well, and drink lots of water.

Key Workout: Tennis—especially if you have a cute outfit and play doubles.

2010 Saturn enters your sign and you're going to work hard, my friend. Career,
health, friends, home, love—you name it, it's time for *Extreme Makeover:*
Upgrade Edition. If something isn't right, the stars say fix it. Conserve your
energy, don't delay what you can do today, and embrace change.

Key Workout: Soft-lit yoga classes.

2011 As you continue your hard work on life improvement, energy moves into
your house of love, partnership, and winning wars. If you need new love, it's
yours. If you want renewed romance, you've got it. But you can't hide in
someone's arms forever. Stay focused on your goals.

Key Workout: One-on-one Pilates instruction.

Signs of Life

Although you are always and forever a Libra, you do have little sweet and sour bits
that don't always fit your peace-loving mold. You know that there are times when
you sink a little bit more into indulgence or when you need to be alone so badly you
could smack someone. There's good reason for this. Read the following signs for
clues to different parts of your life. You're not out of balance; you're interesting.

Love life—Aries

Career—Cancer

Flirtation—Aquarius

Health—Pisces

scorpio-action

THE SCORPION October 23–November 21

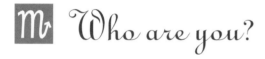

In One Word: INTENSE

Symbol(s): The Scorpion, a shy, private creature with a thin shell for protection, harmless until threatened, then deadly.

Colors: Black and red

Element: WATER. Scorpio is the second of three water signs, more vulnerable than Cancer but also more intense. Scorpio is an extreme sign—emotionally, psychically, and spiritually. Water conducts so much powerful information and energy in this sign that most Scorpios have to limit their exposure. This is what makes you shy, private, and secretive. Unleashed, the water of Scorpio is the most passionate and sexual of the zodiac.

Energy: FIXED. Do not tell a Scorpio what to do or risk being annihilated. It's a simple fact but the world won't learn this lesson. You decide how and when you'll move, and when disturbed, you lash out. Your deadly tail will sting when you feel invaded. As hard as it is to share your needs, it's best to warn others when you're not going to listen to them.

Psychic Domain: Scorpio rules sex, death, and transformation. That explains why the sign is so intense. Of course, Scorpios love sex (in French, the orgasm is called "le petit mort" or "the little death") and all the passion and intensity leading up to it. Ironically, Scorpios find intimacy difficult because it means exposing private, sacred information with someone else. Trust doesn't come easily. Scorpio is perhaps the most complicated, creative, and extreme sign of the zodiac. You're not easy, but you're worth it.

Physical Domain: Where else? Your private parts. Scorpio rules both the regenerative (reproductive) and degenerative (excretory) organs of the body. We don't freely discuss these physical areas and Scorpios prefer it that way.

What to Avoid in the Scorpio Workout: Anything that lacks intensity.

Ideal Workout: Exercise that involves extreme effort, including ballet, long-distance running, weight-lifting, triathlons, and any other sport that requires you to push yourself and hit a new mark. Scorpio is a little bit like Aries, the sign that loves a challenge, although it's not the ability to conquer that Scorpio craves, it's about getting there under duress. An easy target would be way too dull—if a three-mile run gets your heart going, a half-mile sprint at the end is the Scorpio equivalent to heaven. However, you don't need to do extreme sports to feel that intense satisfaction.

Essential Workout Gear: Clothes with body-skimming, weightless stretch.

Ultimate Trouble Spot: Upper arms.

Workout Buddy Warning: First of all, you are not someone who needs a workout buddy. Second, if you do choose to work out with someone, make sure your buddy knows you can be difficult and can forgive you for it. Third, you'll be hard pressed to find someone up for your degree of intensity. In other words, unless it's your sister (or someone who understands your moods and won't be offended by them), don't work out with a buddy.

If You Have a Personal Trainer:

1. You need someone who uses few words and chooses those words carefully. He or she must never use the words *gentle, low-impact, easy,* or *light* to describe a training session, which are all highly unmotivating for a Scorpion. And, at any rate, a chatty sort will turn you off completely.

2. Your trainer should have intense sexual appeal/appetite/drive, guaranteed to produce an instant kinship between the two of you.

3. Make sure your trainer doesn't ask too many personal questions. You hate intrusion.

Strategic Choices for Scorpio

The Scorpio Diet: As a lover of extremes, Scorpio can be a very binge/purge sign. You might have extreme preferences as a kid like sweets, hot chilies, and garlic, but as you get older you learn moderation by watching others, and you try to avoid deprivation and total gorging. It's not so much about what you eat but how much and when you consume. The great strength of Scorpio is that you can put yourself on the most extreme diet and stick to it as long as it takes. The same strength can keep you in a vicious cycle of overeating—and you won't quit until you are good and ready. You're not one to listen to a nutritionist, doctor, or even your mom. Any changes you make need to come from some kind of personal revelation.

Emotional eating is very Scorpion. Feeling low, insecure, or depressed can make you place a chair in front of your fridge until you've cleaned it out. Opting for exercise instead of food is a great way to channel that internal frustration into something healthy. Water signs tend to like alcohol, which can lead Scorpio to trouble because your love of intensity can express itself through overdrinking. This will stress your entire digestive tract as well as put weight on where you don't need it.

The hardest thing for the passionate, intense Scorpio is moderation. On the surface, moderation sounds pathetic, unattractive, and boring. But when you're enjoying in moderation things you like (chocolate, alcohol, pizza, spaghetti, tacos, etc.) you get what you want and look great too. Taking smaller portions of all the things you love doesn't deprive you of pleasure; it just makes it less toxic.

Because of your reactive ways with food, Scorpios can benefit greatly with a few simple dining habits. First, never keep food in plain sight. Structure your kitchen so everything has its own place in the cupboards, drawers, and fridge. When you walk into your kitchen all you want to see are the stove, sink, and a dishtowel or two. Second, turn your pantry (if you have one) into extra storage space or a laundry room. Scorpios shouldn't "stock up" on Doritos, Pop-Tarts, or spaghetti. This stuff just becomes fodder for extreme eating. Third, toss out or regift the lovely gifts of food you receive. It may seen ungrateful, but you've got to turn your back on the neighbor's baked batch of cookies, a coworker's box of chocolates, even that distant relative who mails you a fruitcake every Christmas—get these thoughtful, calorie-laden sweets out of reach immediately. To a Scorpion, these gifts have potential to ruin a day, like rain ruins a picnic.

THE TOP THREE ITEMS TO SHOP FOR:

1. **Cajun spices, like paprika, allspice, sage, chili powder.** You're spicy and you like your food to be too. These spices are healthy because they help increase blood circulation, eradicate sinus congestion, and provide a swift stimulation to the mind and body safely. Sprinkle as a garnish, season meat, mix into dressings and soups. Spices like these add flavor and aroma to just about everything, in a Scorpion snap . . . without added fat or calories, and they'll help you slow down when you eat too.

2. **Cranberry juice.** Since you are extra conscious of the goings-on in your pelvic region, keep your GI tract infection-free by drinking diluted cranberry juice—half juice, half filtered water. Make sure that it's real cranberry juice, and not the "high fructose corn syrup with cranberry flavoring" kind.

3. **Dark chocolate.** Proven to be a mood enhancer, packed with antioxidants, dark chocolate is healthy chocolate.

Diet Vice: Extreme anything.
Signature Spa Treatment: Brazilian bikini wax.
Complementary Therapy: Past-life regressions.
Mindfulness Mantra: It is safe to share my creativity with the world.

Scorpio is such a powerful, creative, and passionate sign, it's almost too much for any one person to handle. That's why you want to hide so much of what you have going on inside. It's almost easier to pretend to be someone else or to act like someone you're not. Many of the great movie actresses are Scorpios: Julia Roberts, Meg Ryan, Toni Colette, and Winona Ryder to name a few. Your ability to feel deeply and bring intense creative energy to whatever you do is a real gift. Of course, to fulfill all that promise you have to actually trust that the world wants what you have to give. We do! And you have to believe that you won't be hurt. Because this is impossible, you might not take the risks you need to for success. Scorpio has a long rule book for "How the World Should Behave." Unfortunately, you never let anyone read it. So how are we supposed to know what to do? Be as generous with forgiveness as you'd like others to be for you and all will go in your favor.

Scorpio in a Nutshell

MIND: Sharp, penetrating, focused, with an extensive catalogue of grudges and distrusts, your mind is an archive of information that needs to be cleaned out now and then. You don't often rely on logic to make decisions but if you did, you'd be just fine. Once you focus on what you want to do or learn, it's as good as done. So focus on the positive and you'll be living the high life.

BODY: Scorpios need only a body as a tool to feel bliss. You love those high notes—extra endorphins, a third glass of wine, amazing passion, or an extra hour of sleep. But your body needs some normal time too. It's a challenge for Scorpios to find happiness in a normal range of emotion but you can do it, especially when you focus on your fuel and fitness. You won't crave more when you feel content with what you have.

SPIRIT: You hold the seeds of all creativity. Grow them with love and reap a harvest of fulfillment.

Allow yourself to express who you are in its truest form.
Let the world reflect your beauty back to you.

A Scorpio Workout Story

Scorpion Cathy wasn't the least bit athletic until she started dating Marco, the cyclist. A little background on Marco . . . he was raised Christian, loves Jesus, worships road-racing. For their one-year anniversary as a couple, Marco gave Cathy a very high-end bike, with a matching (aerodynamic) helmet and a pair of those fancy cycling shoes that click into the pedals, "making the rider one with the bike." At first, Cathy thought, *Wow, what a great gift.* After all, Marco had basically invited her into his sacred space—the cycling world—a huge step in their relationship. Soon after, on their first bike-date, Cathy hit a major pothole. She realized that "cycling" wasn't the same as "riding a bike."

Oh, did she have a lot to learn. Her form was bad and her alignment was off... AND, at the end of their debut ride, Cathy lost her balance, didn't "click out" of the pedals fast enough, and ended up kissing the pavement instead of Marco. Her knee was skinned and her ego was bruised. Three months went by, and the spiffy bike, matching helmet, and fancy shoes stayed in the garage, teetering against the recycling bin.

Then, on a random Tuesday, without goading from Marco, and without any seemingly significant event, Cathy woke up and decided to get back in the saddle again, gearing up and riding into a brisk winter dawn. The moral of the story is this: Yes, Scorpios are physically tough, but they are very easily psyched-out. A lot goes on inside The Scorpion mind. It wasn't the physical challenge of cycling that frightened Cathy as much as the mental strife that went on inside her head.

Marco (obviously a pro at dealing with Cathy) didn't intrude or confront her about her riding ordeal. He granted her the time and space to recover on her own terms. Bravo, Marco! And we're happy to report that today Cathy considers herself a cyclist. (She's got a tight tush to prove it!)

THE SCORPIO "INTENSE PEAK" WORKOUT

Scorpios need to be challenged, and go to their limit, but they also must avoid exhaustion. They need to find intensity without boring repetition or an extreme duration. Unlike earth sign Capricorn, for Scorpio the two-hour workout session is never necessary, unless she's in training for the Tour de France.

What's a Scorpion girl to do? Use that powerful focus to perfect your fitness through an interval *Intense Peak Workout.* We'll keep your heart going pitter-patter throughout this 42-minute total body conditioning routine by blending plyometrics, weight training with low reps, heavy-ish free weights, and standing-core stimulators. Because of its blended nature, the Scorpion workout is not divided into three official parts. Instead, it's one big sequence of exercises to be repeated five times through, followed by a breath-focused one-minute cooldown. You'll stick with each exercise for fifty seconds with ten seconds in transition before moving on to the next exercise. After five circuits you'll chill down your sweaty body for two minutes, and then head off to the shower.

Every exercise is performed from a standing position, so you'll never need a mat. A stopwatch may be helpful, however. Put on some rockin' tunes, move from exercise to exercise at a swift pace, and put your all into every nanosecond. Be sure to wear supportive footwear because there are some high impact moves in your routine. Use a heavy set of free weights (8–10 lb each). No need to count reps either. Just do your best for fifty seconds at each interval, take your time during the ten-second intermission, then buckle down and go for it again.

THREE WORKOUT GOALS FOR SCORPIO

1. Keep your body cleansed with routines that make you sweat.

2. Align your chakras to stay in balance.

3. Let yourself escape as you work out.

WORKOUT PRESCRIPTION

Consistency wins the race, so avoid a workout-feast or a workout-famine. Aim for five workout days per week with two days off. When you strike a good balance in one area of your life, you'll be surprised to see how other areas become steadier as well. You don't have to be competitive or be a "natural" at some sport, you only have to want to learn or participate and you'll get there. Best not to glance around to see who's better. You're not motivated by competition, anyway. You're motivated by what makes you feel great. Find your thing—barre classes, modern dance, squash, swimming—and you'll enjoy building your strength and seeing your body shift.

On a final note, make sure your workout level is intense enough to produce endorphins. Of course, endorphins feel good to everybody, but for a Scorpio, the rush is extra euphoric and thus, extra motivating.

BEST TIME TO WORK OUT: Late morning or noon.

STEP 1: Circuit.

Lateral Jump

(PLYOMETRIC)

Stand with feet together, core muscles activated, and arms by your sides. Bend your knees and tilt your upper body forward slightly, in preparation for a jump.

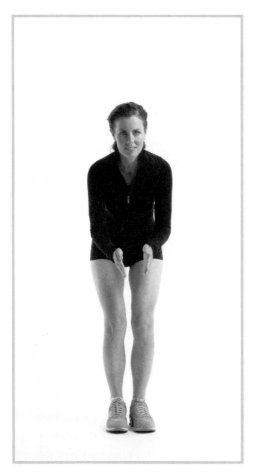 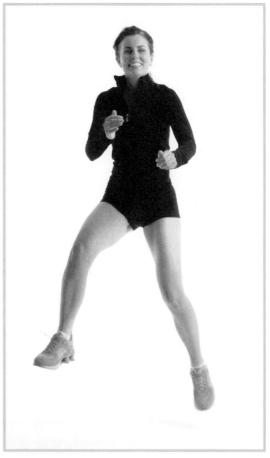

Strongly and aggressively push off the ground and "leap" to the right. Land with slightly bent knees, and then with that same energy, "leap" to the left. Alternate from side to side for fifty seconds. Return to the starting position between leaps.

Overhead Triceps Dip

(STRENGTH TRAINING)

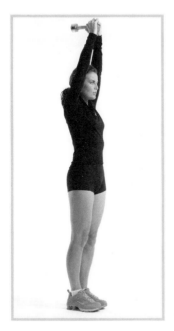 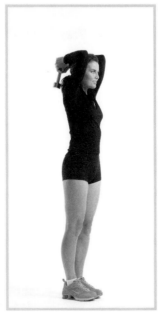

Grab your handheld weight and stand with your feet together and arms together overhead.

With abs in, bend and straighten the elbows in a fluid, up-tempo, controlled manner. Perform as many repetitions as possible in a fifty second time frame. Then carefully drop the weight and proceed to the next exercise.

The Rocket

(PLYOMETRIC)

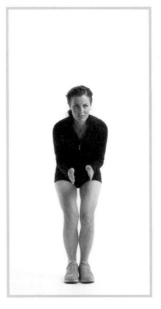 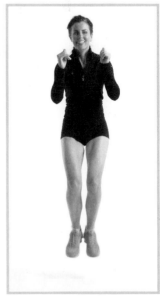

Stand with feet together, core muscles activated, and arms by your sides. Bend both knees and tilt the upper body forward slightly, in preparation for the jump.

With plenty of vigor, jump straight up, like a rocket. Get as much flight as you possibly can, then land with knees slightly bent. Repeat ambitiously for fifty seconds.

Side Arm Circle

(STRENGTH TRAINING)

Grab your weights, and plant your feet in parallel, about six inches apart. Extend your arms out like airplane wings, at shoulder level, holding one weight in each hand. Circle both arms simultaneously in a clockwise rotation, making circles about the size of a salad plate. After approximately twenty-five seconds (the halfway point), reverse direction and rotate counterclockwise. Once the full fifty seconds are over, put down the weights and proceed to the next exercise.

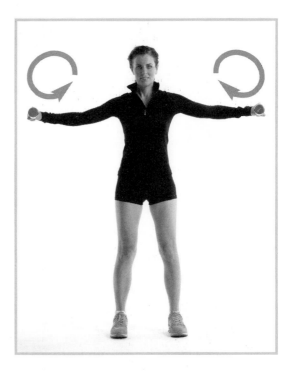

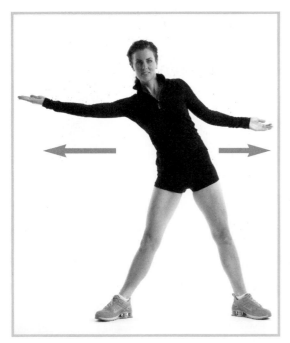

Rib Cage Reaches

(CORE CONDITIONING)

Stand with feet together, core muscles activated, and arms slightly extended out to the sides with palms facing up. From the waist, without moving the hips, reach to the right and then the left from the waist, stretching and squeezing the obliques along the side body. Repeat mindfully and in complete control for fifty seconds, alternating right and left.

Jump Squat

(PLYOMETRIC)

This exercise resembles a jumping jack performed in slow motion. Start standing with arms by your sides, abs in. Bend both knees slightly and lean the torso forward, placing your palms on your thighs.

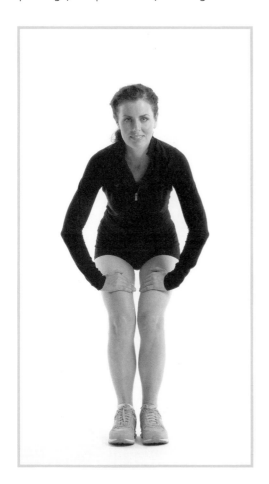
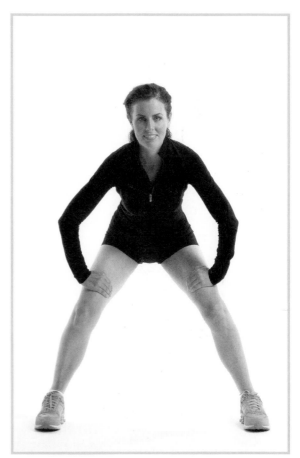

Simply jump wide, into a low squat. Plant the feet firmly as you land. Jump back up to standing and again plant the feet firmly on the landing. Repeat at an ambitious tempo for fifty seconds.

The Heave-Ho

(STRENGTH TRAINING)

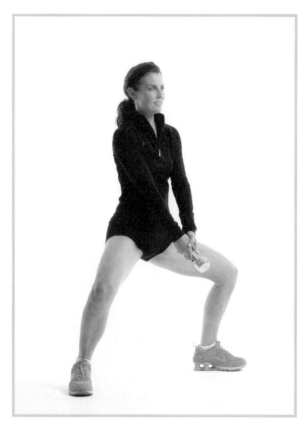

Grab your weight in both hands. Stand with feet apart, abdominals activated. Your weight is at waist level, directly in front of you to start.

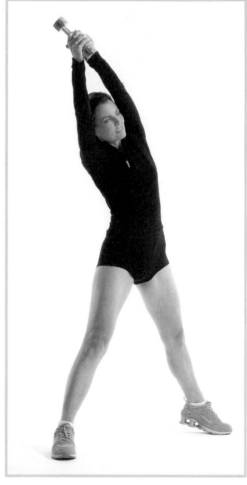

With complete control, bring the weight up and over to the right, without bending the elbows. Bring weight back to starting position, then "heave-ho" the weight up and over to the left, without bending the elbows. Keep alternating in a smooth, steady fashion for fifty seconds. Put down the weight and move on to the next exercise.

Windshield Wiper Kick

(CORE CONDITIONING)

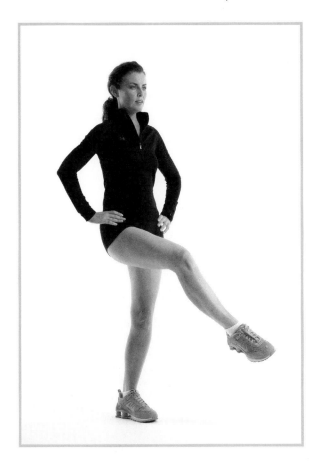

Stand tall with hands at waist, abdominals engaged.

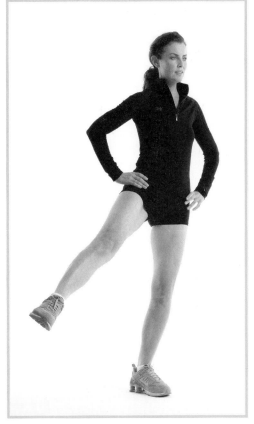

Kick the right leg up as high as it can go (without compromising your tall posture), then sweep it out away from body. Immediately plant the right foot and kick the left leg up. Alternate side to side in a controlled fashion for fifty seconds.

129

STEP 2: Cooldown: Breathing Body (Part 1), Breathing Arms (Part 2). Here is a great way to cool down.

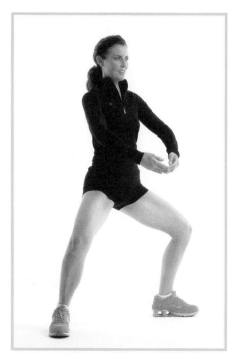

Breathing Body

Begin by using your entire body for breathing. Start with an exhale, knees bent, arms down, then inhale as the knees straighten and the arms go up overhead. Do four reps.

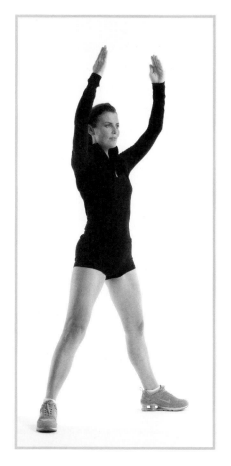

Breathing Arms

Then stand tall and move just the arms up with each inhale and down with each exhale, again four times. Then after you've performed a total of eight, stand and simply breathe without using the arms or the legs. This cooldown will take approximately one minute. Try to slow the breath down and linger at the top of the inhale and at the bottom of the exhale.

What's Ahead of Scorpio: A Star-Driven Five-Year Plan

2007   Coming off a year of opened doors and new experiences, you're ready to settle down and make some money. Optimism and excitement are high on your emotional list so make the most of this happy year. Get out and try a new sport while you have the energy and positive attitude.
Key Workout: What haven't you done? Rock climbing? Cross-country skiing? Maybe gyrotonics?

2008   Energy shifts into more cerebral places. You feel the pull of your lair, your cave. Privacy is at a premium, though, so make the most of your workout time to give you that internal space you crave. You can be a social success and still find time to be a loner.
Key Workout: Long walks with your iPod, lap swimming.

2009   Too many people around you is tough to handle and you may well do some friendship triage to make it easier on yourself. Your home life beckons and your kitchen is begging for attention. Cooking for yourself, working out with friends: that's the recipe for balance this year.
Key Workout: Paddle tennis.

2010   Planets add a new level of flirtation to your life and you'll come crawling out of your hole more often now. Your secretive love life might cause you anxiety, though, so try to find ways to feel more trusting and open. Find your inner goddess with some challenging exercises.
Key Workout: African dance classes, striptease workouts, or Kundalini Yoga.

2011   Planets still emphasize love and commitment while at the same time pushing your privacy buttons and keeping your pretty face out of sight. Balance love and seclusion with good, strong energy. Get outside as much as possible and get your rest. Simple, but not so easy.
Key Workout: Hiking with your boyfriend.

zodiaction

Signs of Life

Scorpio might be the most extreme sign of the zodiac but you sure aren't boring. Your life isn't just about gusto and intensity. You have more to you than that. Here's a little glimpse of how other signs inform different aspects of your life. Yes, Scorpio is your default button, but you do have other vibes.

Love life—Taurus

Career—Leo

Flirtation—Pisces

Health—Aries

sagittarius-action

THE ARCHER November 22–December 21

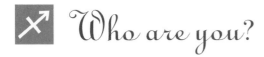 *Who are you?*

In One Word: ADVENTUROUS

Symbol(s): The Archer, half man, half horse, traversing the sky with a bow and arrow. The Archer seeks adventure, experience, and knowledge. When he rests, he shares his thoughts with us.

Color: Twilight blue

Element: FIRE. Sagittarius is the last of the three fire signs. Where Aries is Warrior and Leo is King, Sagittarius is the Court's Advisor, a Merlin. The overarching energy of Sagittarian fire tries to see the world from the height of the sky. Sagittarian fires light up wisdom and bring new cultural understanding and new philosophies to the world.

Energy: MUTABLE. The Archer's head is easily turned in new directions. Sagittarius combines the combustibility of fire with the shiftiness of mutable energy. It's a challenge to get anything done because the world is such an interesting place. This mutable energy makes Sagittarius resilient, however, as well as affable. Sagittarians make friends easily but often don't pay enough attention to them as they move on to more interesting grounds.

zodiaction

Psychic Domain: Sagittarius is the philosopher, the risk-taker, and the joyful truth-teller of the zodiac. Sagittarians are generally lucky since Jupiter, the planet of luck, rules the sign. Sagittarius oversees large-scale information like film, publishing, television, and the news media. You're someone who does not shy away from saying what's on your mind. Sagittarians are known for being "painfully honest" or "frank to a fault." San Mateo–based astrologer Susan Strong attributes this to the fact that "what's in your mind comes out your mouth," without time to edit.

Physical Domain: Since The Archer needs power in his legs to leap through the sky, Sagittarius rules the thighs, hips, and sciatic nerve. Your ruler, Jovial Jupiter, loves to enjoy himself. That makes Sagittarians good-time girls, especially when it comes to good food. Jupiter is an expanding energy and a Sagittarian needs to keep an eye on those thighs and that waistline to make sure Jupiter isn't having *too* good a time.

What to Avoid in the Sagittarius Workout: Static, repetitive anything.

Ideal Workout: Fitness is another frontier for the adventurous Sagittarian, but you need to go somewhere to practice your art, or learn something new in order for your mutable energy to stay tuned. Exercise needs to have a point—conditioning for a long-distance bike trip, getting in shape for a horse show, running along a safe path under an evening sky. You are the worst candidate for day-in, day-out routine. You need variation, changing scenery, and a reason to go.

Essential Workout Gear: Lycra bottoms, comfy tops. Cross-trainers.

Ultimate Trouble Spot: Thighs.

Workout Buddy Warning: If you choose to work out with someone else, they'd better be interesting. No sissies, wussies, or whiners. You do like company but not enough to put up with tedious conversation. Besides, your inability to look interested when you're not won't help you in the end, unless you want to let this person know they're on your "out" list.

If You Have a Personal Trainer:

1. You need an adventurous, can-do personality.

2. Your trainer should be heavily built.

3. You need a highly knowledgeable trainer who brings you lots of advice and information you can use. He/she should be like a sports-conditioning coach.

Strategic Choices for Sagittarius

The Sagittarian Diet: Adventure, experience, and a willingness to try new things is the Sagittarian prescription. You're not shy of foreign foods, even if they do incorporate ingredients that evoke fear in others. When you find something you like, you enjoy it. Otherwise, you move on. The Sagittarian's diet isn't so much about what you eat—it's about how much.

Sagittarius is an enthusiastic sign, which is why you often find yourself overdoing it with favorite foods. And since variety is the spice of life, Sagittarians have a lot of favorites. Whether it's a hot Indian curry or a Thai BBQ, you're up for it—and your weight might be too.

There are two devils for the Sagittarian watching her weight and waistline. The first is lingering. There's nothing more fun than sitting around a good meal with good wine and good friends, enjoying the atmosphere and conversation at a leisurely pace. While others push back plates and sip water after wine, the Sagittarian will haplessly take another glass or absentmindedly pick the crumbs off her neighbor's dessert plate. The second devil is the "on-the-run" diet, where nutrition is a quick fix between jobs or dates. The busy and adventurous Sagittarian won't stop to think about fat grams or sugar content. If you're hungry and it's there, you'll grab it so you can get on with your project. Planning ahead (like packing Ziploc baggies with carrot sticks) isn't your forte. That's just the way it is.

Lean into high protein over carbs. And go with the five little meals instead of three squares so that you always feel full and aren't tempted to overeat.

Sagittarians can eat almost *anything.* You just have to be careful not to eat almost *everything.*

THE TOP THREE ITEMS TO SHOP FOR:

1. **Pre-washed salad mixes sold in bulk or bags.** You aren't into preparing this stuff, so it's best to buy it ready-to-go.

2. **Individually packaged low-fat yogurt.** Healthy, high-protein, portion-controlled, portable snacks.

3. **Dry roasted or raw pumpkin seeds (also called *pepitas* in Spanish).** Pumpkin seeds are commonly eaten as a nutritious snack or added to casseroles, salads, and

bread. High in omega-3 fatty acids, along with a high concentration of protein and zinc, they are a bull's-eye for The Archer's energy needs.

Diet Vice: Seconds.

Signature Spa Treatment: Steam room or sauna.

Complementary Therapy: Cleansing fast.

Mindfulness Mantra: Life offers adventure in every moment.

Sagittarius is an expansive, generous, and jovial sign. Most Sagittarians are positive people with curious, let's-take-a-shot attitudes. You're good at a party, interested in learning and trying new things, and you aren't afraid to explore relationships when they hit your passion play button. Your energy is refreshing and alive when you're happy and healthy. When you're tired or anxious, you could seem rash, braggy, or simply tough. You don't have an automatic shut-off system; instead, you lose your softness and can turn abrasive or inattentive. Your head can turn too quickly! Sagittarians tell the truth no matter what, but you don't always think about your audience before proclaiming the bare facts. It's your spiritual purpose to be honest, but you don't have to be brutal. You can be sensitive when you want to be, so don't downplay others' emotions. When you're healthy and clearheaded, there is no one better to be around.

Sagittarius in a Nutshell

MIND: Quick, engaged, and a great student when you're interested—Sagittarians love to think, feel, explore, and intuit information. Whether you're learning about foreign cultures or taking classes from a shaman, you're all about experiencing things firsthand. You're sporty, charming, and witty and you forgive easily—a great gift.

BODY: As you leap across the universe your powerful legs propel you. Don't get caught up in trying to be stick-thin. It's not healthy for any Sagittarius to forgo muscle. You're the picture of health and balance: muscular strength, powerhouse curves, and agile, flexible joints. Embrace your vitality.

SPIRIT: You enlighten and enliven. The seeds of knowledge are spread through your explorations.

Seek knowledge both inside yourself and out in the world.
Allow your inner truth to speak with compassion and integrity.

A Sagittarius Workout Story

Jessica has always been plagued with tight hamstrings. Even in grade school ("the flexible years") she couldn't bend down to touch her toes. For years she chalked it up to genetics and avoided yoga, Pilates, and painting her own toenails. Instead she opted to master the sport of golf. Fair enough. Golf is a great sport for Sagittarius—social, outdoors, mentally challenging.

However, the time came when Jessica could ignore her Achilles' heel no more, when those tight hamstrings affected her progress on the green. She actually had to withdraw from a few tournaments due to a chronic pull. Sags abhor sitting on the sideline—you want to play the game! Jess hit an all-time low.

Desperate times call for desperate measures, so Jess enrolled in a series of Pilates classes. Yes, they were torture, especially in the beginning, when the instructor showed little compassion. Pilates wasn't just challenging and uncomfortable, it downright hurt! But since her golf game depended on a bit more flexibility, she stuck with it. Sometimes what you want to do the *least* is what your body needs the *most*.

Can Jessica touch her toes now? Nope, but that wasn't the goal. The goal was to improve her hamstring situation and make her way back to the course. *Zodiaction* is happy to report that Jessica is back to driving, putting, and teeing off—Sag success.

THE SAGITTARIUS "ZEST FOR LIFE" WORKOUT

Sagittarians need to get up and get out in any workout. As a thrill-seeking, risk-taking sign, though, you need to maintain some sort of plan. There's no point in pushing yourself into injury or danger, so set goals—maybe at two or three levels so that you have the thrill of going "beyond," but don't get carried away.

zodiaction

1. *Exhilarating Cardio* that'll burn calories and fat.

2. *Total Body Boot Camp* that'll tone and tighten all over.

3. *Super Stretch* that'll release tension and improve flexibility.

All three components require no equipment and can be performed anywhere, on a mountaintop, at the beach, or in your hotel room.

THREE WORKOUT GOALS FOR SAGITTARIUS

1. Keep yourself balanced and focused with stretching. You struggle to see the reason for stretching—but trust us when we say stretch to prevent injury, to increase your range of motion, and to soothe muscles after a workout.

2. Rotate through a variety of cardio workouts so you don't get bored. Cardio, cardio, cardio—you love it, you need it, and you'll find it everywhere you look.

3. You tend to get very sports-specific, which is great, but be careful to work out off the course/court/slope every week. Sports alone tend to cause muscular imbalance, which, over time, can cause misalignment and lead to a chronic injury.

WORKOUT PRESCRIPTION

Sagittarius has needs. First, you need to have fun. Forget the treadmill and other cardio equipment in your gym—they embody the *Sagittarian three strikes:* they're indoors, non-social, and stationary. Second, you need to incorporate flexibility training. Force yourself to stretch every day. Third, you need to be active every single day. This activity doesn't have to be a formal workout. It could be a brisk walk to work, a swing dance session, or a game of tag with your nieces.

BEST TIME TO WORK OUT: Daytime—whenever the mood strikes.

STEP 1: Exhilarating Cardio. The Sagittarian's cardiovascular experience should provoke a feeling of freedom in the great outdoors. Hiking, running, skiing, canoeing, and cycling are perfect choices for you, rain or shine. Just make sure you have quality gear, be it a bike, boots, or a bra. The right stuff will keep your mind on the exhilaration rather than a potential malfunction. Aim for thirty to sixty minutes of heart-pumping training. Get sweaty. Deeply heat your muscles. Then move on to Step 2.

STEP 2: Total Body Boot Camp. Now that you're breathing big, let's venture directly into strength training. Big ranges of motion mix with your own body weight for a boot-camp experience. Access your signature Sagittarian pep and work these exercises like Rocky.

Walking Lunges

(TONES THE MUSCLES OF THE LEGS AND PROVIDES A SUBTLE BALANCE CHALLENGE)

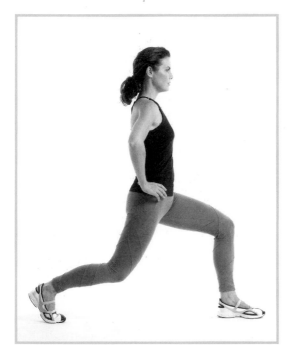

Step your left leg forward, keeping your torso upright. The back heel should be lifted off the ground. Engage your core muscles and be sure to have both feet pointing straight ahead.

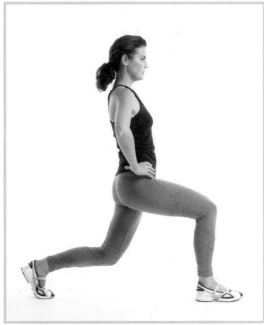

Keep your torso erect and generously step the right foot forward, in a "walking" lunge. Alternate left then right for a total of ten repetitions.

zodiaction

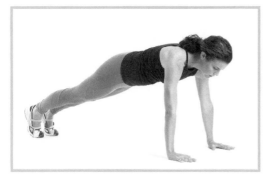

Knee Cross Crunch

(TONES THE MUSCLES OF THE CORE)

Begin in Plank position with the palm of each hand placed directly underneath each shoulder. The abdominals should be pulled in and the spine (including the neck) should be in one fairly straight line.

Exhale and squeeze the left knee up toward the right shoulder. Immediately switch, and bring the right knee to the left shoulder. Alternate for a total of twenty repetitions.

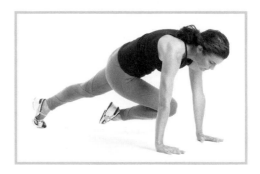

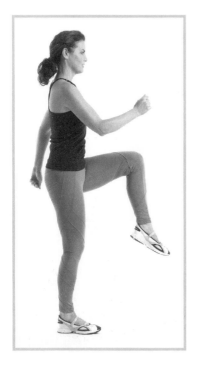

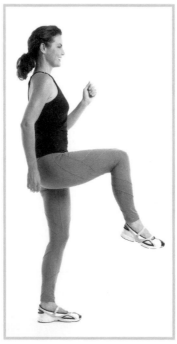

Knee-Ups

(TONES THE MUSCLES OF THE CORE AND INCREASES THE HEART RATE FOR AN EXCELLENT CARDIOVASCULAR CHALLENGE)

Stand tall, engage your core muscles, and bring your left knee up to the chest.

Quickly (and with a slight "bounce") switch and bring your right knee up to the chest. Repeat for a total of fifty quick alternating Knee-Ups.

Wide Stance Push-Up

(TONES THE MUSCLES OF THE UPPER BODY)

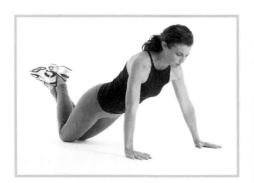

Place the palms of your hands approximately six inches wider than shoulder-distance apart. Bend your knees and cross your ankles.

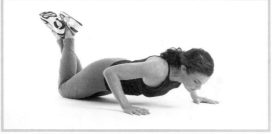

Bend and straighten the elbows in a swift, smooth movement, without disturbing the body's alignment. Repeat fifteen times at a brisk and even tempo.

Single Straight Leg Crunch

(A VERY CHALLENGING ABDOMINAL STRENGTHENER)

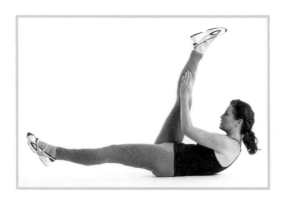

Lie on your back with chin in toward your chest and shoulder blades off the floor. Grab hold of your right leg and bring it up toward the ceiling. Keep your legs straight and point your toes.

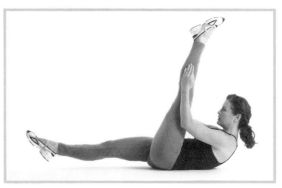

Exhale, scissor the legs, and grab hold of the left leg. Scissor and switch again. Keep alternating for a full set of twenty repetitions.

Hip Lift

(AN EXCELLENT ABDOMINAL STRENGTHENER)

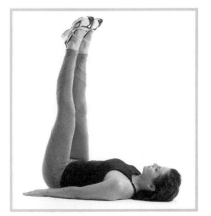

Lie on your back with the head and shoulders resting comfortably on the floor. Extend both legs straight up, forming an "L" with your body. Arms are at your sides.

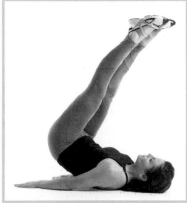

Exhale, squeeze the navel toward the spine, and lift the hips up off the floor. Inhale and return the hips to the floor. Repeat for a total of twenty repetitions.

STEP 3: Super (Duper) Stretch. Learn to love it, Sag! Stretching is your gateway to new frontiers, plus it'll help prevent injury. Here we hold each stretch for an honest sixty seconds.

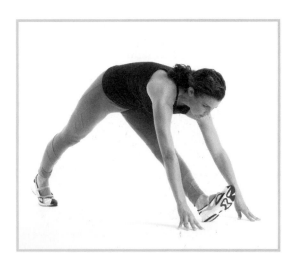

The Teeter Totter

(A VERY CHALLENGING HAMSTRING STRETCH)

This exercise is performed standing with the torso leaning forward. Begin with the legs apart in a straddle, keeping both legs straight. Lift toe of the front foot and heel of back foot off the floor. Place your hands on either side of the front leg for balance. Hold for sixty seconds, and then repeat with the other leg forward.

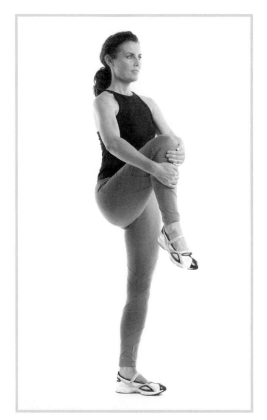

Standing
Knee to Chest

(IMPROVES BALANCE WHILE STRETCHING THE BUTTOCK AND LOWER BACK MUSCLES)

Stand tall, grab hold of your knee, and hug it in toward your chest. Balance there for sixty seconds and then switch legs.

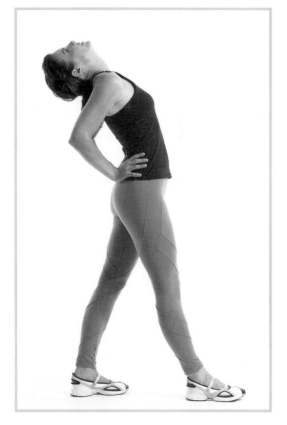

Standing Back Bend

(IMPROVES THE RANGE OF MOTION OF THE SPINE)

Stand tall, with one foot in front of the other for balance, and place your hands on your lower back. Lift your chest up toward the sky and arch backward. Allow your head to drop back as well. Be sure to keep your eyes open. Hold for sixty seconds.

Seated Straddle

(STRETCHES THE INNER THIGHS AND HAMSTRINGS)

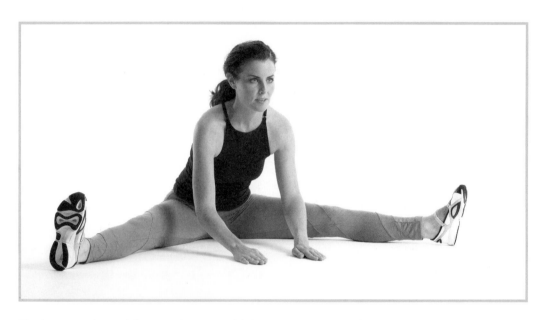

Sit down and straddle your legs as widely as you can comfortably go. Maintain straight legs if possible. Now simply lean forward, resting your upper body weight upon your hands. Hold for sixty seconds.

What's Ahead of Sagittarius: A Star-Driven Five-Year Plan

2007   There's no denying this is a year of opportunity, luck, and adventure. Your ruler leaps through your sign with enthusiasm and vitality. Can you make the best of the choices you encounter? Sure you can. Just remember to choose healthy eating while you're at it.
Key Workout: Set a new goal for your mile time.

2008   Hard work and career achievement are highlighted while your ruler has you making and spending money as fast as you can. You need as much focus as you can muster. Keep your eyes on your goal and don't be daunted by challenges. You're great at problem-solving.
Key Workout: Racquetball.

2009   The power of communicating with ease and wit is bestowed upon you this
        year. It's a good thing too, because your career issues demand some great
        thinking. Keep stress to a minimum with a smart workout program and when
        in doubt, open a bottle of water instead of a bottle of wine.
        Key Workout: Jogging or power walking.

2010   In a shift of planetary energy, you become more focused on domestic affairs
        than getting out and about. No, it doesn't mean that you'll miraculously
        become a neat freak, but you'll take time to decorate, cook, and just enjoy
        the stuff you've collected over the years. It's nice to sit still once in a while.
        Key Workout: Low-impact, fat-burning workout DVDs.

2011   After a year of rest, you're set to party. Call up the three friends you still care
        about—you are ready for fun. Whether you join a baseball team or
        competitive ballroom dancing, you're prepared for action. You've got a
        sporting advantage this year so you're bound to win.
        Key Workout: Any team sport.

Signs of Life

Sagittarius is an adventurous, curious sign. But you're not always up for a risk or a
challenge. Check out the signs that relate to different parts of your life. Could you be
finicky with career moves and slightly obsessed with your health?

> **Love life**—Gemini
>
> **Career**—Virgo
>
> **Flirtation**—Aries
>
> **Health**—Taurus

capricorn-action

THE GOAT WITH A FISH TAIL December 22–January 19

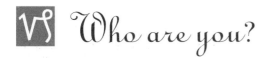

In One Word: ACCOMPLISHED

Symbol(s): Capricorn is usually associated with a goat, animal of tenacity and fortitude, capable of scaling great heights. The fish's tail, an older symbol that has been ignored by some astrological sources, is an important part of Capricorn, as it is the symbol of spiritual connection. Capricorn is the sign that marries our material reality with greater spiritual energy.

Color: Deep forest brown

Element: EARTH. Capricorn is the last of the three earth signs. What Taurus grows, Virgo sorts, and Capricorn then takes over and constructs. Capricorn is the sign that makes this world what it is today and represents all the building it has taken to get here. Capricorn is the power to construct buildings, cities, factories, and industry. It is the most advanced earth form of productivity and progress.

Energy: CARDINAL. With the energy of purpose and accomplishment, Capricorn takes earth energy and directs it toward a goal. Whether this goal is for the greater good or simply for the sake of productivity is up to you. Capricorn cardinal energy can get almost anything done. Hopefully you'll be proud of what you accomplish.

Psychic Domain: You might seem secretive or shy but what you are is dignified. You hold back telling your stories and opinions because you don't want to put yourself "out there" without some reconnaissance. You're the last person who wants a surprise party. You hate being put on the spot until you choose to come forward. You can be quite commanding and you're certainly confident when you feel prepared, but you need to control your environment as much as possible. Capricorn can be accused of being too serious. But when you feel like sharing, no one has a better sense of humor than you.

Physical Domain: Capricorn is about stature and physical reality. It rules the skin, skeletal structure, and more specifically the knees, which are symbolic of authority. You will find that your entire body is sensitive to stress and strain. Skin problems are probably stress-related impurities; aching joints and bones are indicative of heavy burdens. You know when you're overloaded but you can be too stoic. If you have pain, it's time to stop the madness.

What to Avoid in the Capricorn Workout: A plateau. You continuously need new goals.

Ideal Workout: Climbing a mountain. You're the goat, the hiker of the zodiac. Your perfect workout needs an endpoint; whether it's a 3000-ft. peak or a new time on your 5K, you need to hit a mark.

Essential Workout Gear: Orthotics.

Ultimate Trouble Spot: Knees.

Workout Buddy Warning: You need someone who takes things as seriously as you do—or at least someone who can cajole you out of being too serious. It's up to you and your mood. You can appreciate a good sense of humor when you are not being hypersensitive, ultra-competitive, or ridiculously focused on a goal.

If You Have a Personal Trainer:

1. Your trainer should realize that you are already motivated from within, so they need not be too cheerleader-like. Save "good job" and "you can do it" for another client. The Capricorn trainer's dialogue should mostly be about alignment specifics and technique cues.

2. You need a trainer who understands the anatomy of a knee injury and can guide you toward preventing one.

3. Ideally your trainer has achieved a state or national ranking in some sport you respect.

Strategic Choices for Capricorn

The Capricorn Diet: Capricorns are gifted with focus and discipline when you choose to use it. That means you can be totally healthy and careful about your diet. The downside? You're not that into it. You're busy building toward a new goal, not shopping for organic produce. There's not much final satisfaction involved when stocking a fridge and cooking—you only have to do it again and again.

Capricorns are sensitive to the vibes of others and frankly, you worry a lot. You're also prone to hanging with the green-eyed monster, especially when you *perceive* someone to be further along or more accomplished than you. It's a nasty trap, jealousy, and once you fall into negative thinking, your diet goes straight into the garbage. You may not show your emotions to people, but you can easily sublimate them with food.

Capricorns LOVE comfort food and are prone to starch and grease overdosing from time to time. Elvis, a Capricorn born January 8, is a perfect example of this. He too often found comfort in his famous "fried peanut butter and banana sandwiches"! The cheesiest mac & cheese, whipped mashed potatoes, "BBP" ("Big Bowls of Pasta"), or whatever it is that has a security-blanket effect on your psyche, needs to be monitored, or your waistline will suffer. Best not to have these saboteurs in your kitchen. For those times that you must indulge (and we've all got 'em) go out to your favorite diner, sit down, and make a special occasion out of it. You're not a complete pig, of course—that wouldn't be dignified. Just remember that comfort food can wreak havoc, setting you back on your road to accomplishment, so make these carb blowouts an exception rather than a staple.

Like other earth signs, you can be prone to constipation, which can lead to low energy, mega-negativity, and a generally foul mood. Rather than let a little overindulgence get the best of you, find balance in a diet that combines calcium and fiber with energy-boosting foods. Try to keep in mind that food has a direct and instant effect on mood.

THE TOP THREE ITEMS TO SHOP FOR:

1. **Arugula, collard greens, cabbage, or bok choy.** You'll find it easy to create tasty dishes out of these high-fiber, high-calcium greens. Try your hand at a salad or a stew, or a veggie pita sandwich. These foods make for safe grazing too.

2. **Grapefruit.** Lucky us, in this day and age, we can score juicy grapefruits all year long at just about any local market. ~~Try to get~~ Get into the habit of replacing your morning pastry/starch with grapefruit. At first, you'll be kicking and screaming, but once you realize how much cleaner and lighter you feel—and how much more you accomplish—you'll be hooked. (We know you've got the discipline to hang in there and make this a habit.)

3. **Fresh figs.** Figs, fat-free, sodium-free, and cholesterol-free, are a health home run for just about any sign. But what makes figs exceptionally awesome for The Goats of the world is that they possess the highest overall mineral content of all common fruits. A 40 gram ($1/4$ cup) serving provides 244 mg of potassium (7 percent of the DV), 53 mg of calcium (6 percent of the US RDA), and 1.2 mg of iron (6 percent of the US RDA). We want you to ingest plenty of calcium, iron, and potassium for strong blood and bones. Plus, figs are sweet, filling, and can satisfy your "comfort" tooth. (Fig Newtons don't count!)

A final note about the Capricorn diet: It's not about deprivation or eliminating your favorite foods. It's about adding healthy items into your daily eating experience. You're a pretty high-energy sign and you need fuel to climb to the top, be it the corporate ladder, or the mountain peak. Inserting more fiber, more fluid, and more minerals into your diet is going to improve your energy output. You'll live up to your "accomplished" reputation, for sure.

Diet Vice: Diner grub.

Signature Spa Treatment: Full body exfoliation.

Complementary Therapy: Shiatsu.

Mindfulness Mantra: You can accomplish anything with compassion.

Capricorn is a sign that is very self-critical. You always believe that you can do better, be better. You have a lot of goals and you see a lot of potential for reaching them all. Once you do get where you want to be, you set your sights even higher. After all, if you got there, how hard could it have been? You don't give yourself the respect and compassion you deserve.

Your planetary ruler is Saturn, which represents hard work and karma. Being a Capricorn comes with a certain amount of responsibility. You must remember to be compassionate and kind while you accomplish great things. Jesus was a Capricorn (his birthday is December 25) and it has been considered the sign of the Jews as well. Spiritual hard work? You bet.

Capricorn in a Nutshell

MIND: Focused to the point of brooding, your mind is there to serve your need to produce, achieve, and build. If you stay too long in your head, you get depressed. You need to take action toward a goal. Try to set *reasonable* goals, approach them with optimism, and celebrate what you achieve. You can be a great inspirational leader if you stay positive.

BODY: You're pretty in touch with your body. You can't help but notice when your skin is bothering you or your joints ache. The thing to avoid is stoicism. You could fall into that "no pain, no gain" trap and end up ignoring an injury. Respect your limits and you'll get further. You're human and vulnerability comes with the territory.

SPIRIT: You make this world real. Use the energy of spirit to guide you from the heart.

Lead with compassion and the world will follow.
It is profound to appreciate all that you accomplish.

A Capricorn Workout Story

Pilates is a form of fitness in which the details matter. This may explain why Kathleen, a Capricorn hailing from upstate New York, is particularly obsessed with it. Her ability to concentrate at length, paired with her love of doing things properly, make Pilates and Kathleen a marriage made in heaven. She credits Pilates with improving her posture, creating a more flexible lower back, and preserving her youthful appearance.

Iris, a former ballet star with fifteen-plus years of Pilates experience, had been Kathleen's one and only trainer since day one. Iris is "the best, most revered, most experienced trainer," says a low-key Kathleen. This is particularly significant. You see, in true Capricorn fashion, Kathleen has high standards. She wants to be trained by the best, most revered, most experienced trainer or not trained at all.

Then Iris up and moves to Vermont. What's a Goat to do? They get downright bitchy for a while. They trot into the studio with a snobby aura, seemingly unsatisfied with anyone daring to step into Iris's ballet slippers. Watch out world, this negative attitude lingers for a bit. And due to The Goat's discipline and drive, they'll keep showing up for their standing appointments, even though they're dissatisfied with the staff.

It wasn't until one of these replacements, Sophie, wowed Kathleen with a sophisticated cue about keeping the spine "tall like The Statue of Liberty" that she began to respect her new trainer. Things slowly returned to normal. The snotty attitude disappeared and Kathleen was again content while performing *The Hundred*.

(*Trainers:* Beware of the Capricorn curse. Don't take it personally and try to ride it out. *Capricorns:* Keep in mind that you can be intimidating. Try to crack a smile, even if you doubt someone's ability.)

THE CAPRICORN "STEEP AND SCRUPULOUS" WORKOUT

Capricorn needs a real plan that has reachable progress points, anchored by a long-term strategy. You don't need flash. The hottest trend will not appeal to you. You want something that works and works well. And you can do the exact same routine again and again without boredom. Bells and whistles need not apply! All of these Capricorn attributes serve you well in life and on your fitness quest.

Capricorn wants her workout to work. Yes, you're happy with slow and steady results (the more permanent kind), but you need to see and feel authentic results nonetheless. And you want to keep being challenged. A big motivator for you is to be sure that each workout takes you further toward your goal. Here's where you can use your Capricorn patience to build to that goal, be it weight management, muscle tone, or agility.

The Capricorn *Steep and Scrupulous Workout* has two distinct steps. Step 1 is *Steep Cardio*. This is cardiovascular activity that involves an incline. Hiking is ideal. The root action and earthy terrain are appealing to Goats. If you can't get outdoors, the StairMaster and Elliptical machines are the next best things. Treadmills are good too—especially when set to an incline position. Step 2 is *Scrupulous Yogalates* where we are very attentive to detail. In this section we combine seven total body Pilates exercises with five yoga stretches for a smooth, challenging routine that can be performed again and again and again.

The long-range secret weapon within the Capricorn workout is its progression plan. Here we provide you with specific ways you can alter your workout, month by month, in duration, number of repetitions, or intensity. You'll see that there are many possibilities for keeping the challenge alive. Each exercise has four levels to opt from:

A = **Level One.** Perfect for fitness newcomers, postnatal moms, and those returning to fitness after injury. If you choose workout "A," the duration is lower, the intensity is lower, and the number of repetitions is minimum.

B = **Level Two.** Ideal for intermediates. This is the next step for the graduates of "Level One."

C = **Level Three.** Here's a high-intermediate plan that's great for athletes who want to cross-train or for those who simply crave a bigger challenge.

D = **Level Four.** At "D" your duration is longest, the intensity is highest, and the number of repetitions is to the max.

THREE WORKOUT GOALS FOR CAPRICORN

1. Strengthen core muscles without stress on joints.

2. Set up progressive cardio goals and increased levels of difficulty.

3. Keep the legs rejuvenated by inverting them at some point after the cardio climb.

WORKOUT PRESCRIPTION

Accomplishment-oriented Capricorn needs a solid workout program that bows to the holy trinity of strength, tone, and cardio. If your joints are up for it, aim for five days per week. If time is limited, do Step 1 one day, and then Step 2 the next. And, if your knees are aggravating you, it's OK to skip the *Steep Cardio* altogether. Just put some extra zip into your *Scrupulous Yogalates*.

zodiaction

BEST TIME TO WORK OUT: First thing in the morning. Due to your high level of discipline, you may fare well with before-work workouts.

STEP 1: Steep Cardio. The first section for Capricorn is cardio with an incline. This serves two purposes. First, the incline escalates your heart rate into an intense zone **without** having to run, which is very tough on your joints and not a great choice for someone with sensitive knees.

Second, the incline appeals to Capricorn's innate "life is all uphill" disposition. After all, there are always higher levels to strive for.

Do *Steep Cardio* before *Scrupulous Yogalates*. This will warm your body, lubricate your joints, create elasticity in your muscles, and train your lungs to breathe big. Always begin at a strong, yet stable, pace where you establish your rhythm for the entire journey. You'll basically be moving at the same MPH from beginning to end. Over time, your starting pace will become faster and your cardio sessions more intense. You never want to be gasping for air or unable to carry on a conversation. If this is the case, you need to slow down a little bit and connect to your breath. This isn't a walk in the park, nor is it a sprint. It's somewhere in between, with a mission to get fit and stay fit.

Along with intensity, duration plays a key role in your progression plan. For *Steep Cardio,* choose increments of 30, 60, 90, or 120 minutes. If you are super-fit, 30 minutes may seem wimpy. If you're exercise-shy, 120 minutes might seem impossible. But, Capricorn, you are so good with long-term vision. Don't stop before you start! You'll realize no matter what your fitness level is right now, there is a time and a place for all durations; besides, when hiking outside, 120 minutes really does go by in a snap.

Remember, *Steep Cardio* is ultimately about time and intensity. On a scale of one to ten (ten being the most intense) we want you to choose a level eight or nine. Don't get caught up in mileage. When we move at a constant incline, the miles don't really convey the true hard work.

STEP 2: Scrupulous Yogalates. Immediately after your cardio jaunt, clear away some indoor space, kick off your sneakers, and swiftly transition into a stretch/strength mode. Some exercises are yoga poses, while others are Pilates repetitions. All poses and repetitions provide both stretching and strengthening, the two elements necessary to bring your body, mind, and spirit into balance after your hike. We know you like details, so in *Scrupulous Yogalates* we provide acute specifics in order for you to have lots to focus on and work toward.

Eagle Pose
(Garudasana)

*(EAGLE POSE HELPS INCREASE BLOOD FLOW THROUGH THE MAJOR JOINTS OF THE BODY;
THE POSE PROVIDES A GOOD BALANCE CHALLENGE AND A STRETCH TO THE MID AND UPPER BACK MUSCLES)*

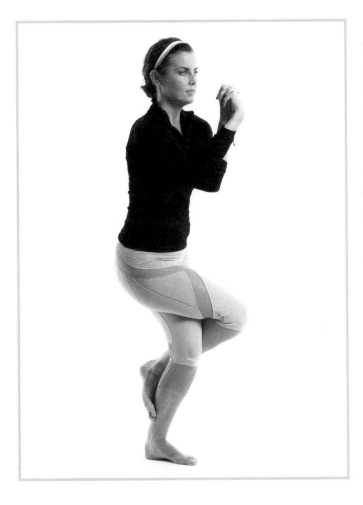

Stand with feet together and arms by your sides. Inhale and lift both arms up overhead. Exhale, bring both arms down, crossing the right arm underneath the left. Interlace your fingers and cross and twist your arms like ropes. Then bend both knees, as if sitting in an invisible chair. Exhale and lift the right leg up and over the left. Cross and twist your legs like ropes. You are now balancing on one leg. Hold for 30 (60, 90, 120) seconds, then repeat once more with the opposite arm and leg on top.

zodiaction

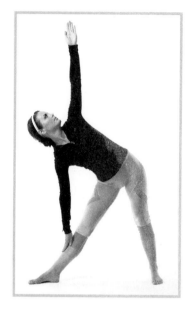

Triangle Pose (Trikonasana)

(THIS YOGA POSE PROVIDES AN EXCELLENT STRETCH TO THE HAMSTRINGS AND INNER THIGH MUSCLES)

Stand with your feet planted approximately four feet apart. Turn your right foot out, so it points away from the body. Turn your left foot in, so it points slightly inward. Both legs remain straight with muscles engaged, and the arms are extended out, like airplane wings. Now windmill the arms down to the right without hunching, and position the right arm lightly upon the right shin. Keep your chest open and look up toward the left thumb. Feel light and lifted as you calmly inhale and exhale. Hold for 30 (60, 90, 120) seconds, then repeat again to the left.

Reverse Plank

(THIS EXERCISE TONES THE ENTIRE CORE AREA, PLUS STRENGTHENS THE THIGHS)

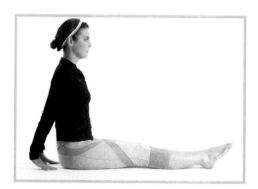

Sit tall with legs extended straight out in front of you. Plant the palms of your hands firmly on the floor just behind you. Engage the muscles of the core.

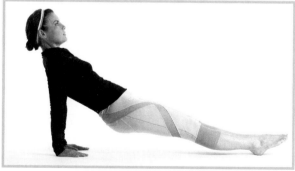

Inhale and with vigor, lift the hips upward, without bending at the spine. Exhale and smoothly return to the starting position. Repeat 5 (10, 15, 20) times total.

Camel Pose (Ustrasana)

(CAMEL IS ONE OF THE BEST CHEST AND ABDOMEN STRETCHES AND MAKES FOR A STRONGER, HEALTHIER BACK TOO)

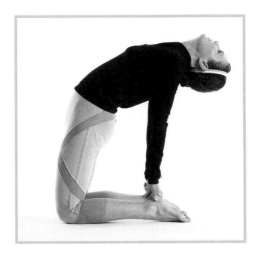

Kneel on the ground with your knees placed approximately six or seven inches apart. Press the palms of your hands into your lower back, with fingers pointing down. Now, cautiously drop your head back, as if getting a shampoo at a salon. As you lift your heart upward, the back arches and the right hand grabs hold of your right heel as the left hand grabs hold of your left heel. Keep your eyes open and your breath calm. Hold for 30 (60, 90, 120) seconds.

One-Legged Bridge

(THIS PILATES EXERCISE TARGETS THE GLUTES AND LOWER BACK EXCEPTIONALLY WELL)

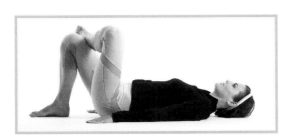

Lie on your back with your head and shoulders comfortably resting upon the floor. Arms relax down by your sides. Plant one foot on the floor and cross the other over the opposite knee.

Exhale and smoothly lift your hips off the floor by articulating the spine one vertebra at a time. When you get to the height of the movement, take an inhalation. Then, just as smoothly, exhale and return to the starting position. Repeat 5 (10, 15, 20) times, then switch legs.

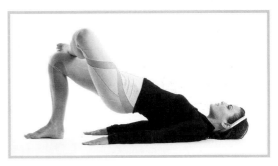

zodiaction

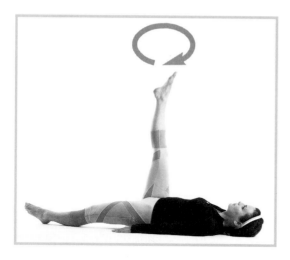

Leg Circle

(THIS PILATES EXERCISE PROVIDES A STRETCHING AND A STRENGTHENING EFFECT FOR THE MUSCLES OF THE THIGHS)

Lie on your back with your head and shoulders comfortably resting upon the floor. Arms relax down by your sides. Extend one leg along the floor and the other straight up toward the ceiling. The knees can bend slightly if necessary, but try to have nice, strong, stretched-out legs. Rotate your leg in a clockwise circle about the size of a dinner plate. Attempt to keep everything else still. Repeat 5 (10, 15, 20) times then reverse directions and rotate counterclockwise for another 5 (10, 15, 20) repetitions. Be sure to switch legs and repeat the whole series once again.

Jackknife

(THIS PILATES EXERCISE IS ONE OF THE ALL-TIME GREATS FOR SIMULTANEOUSLY STRETCHING THE LOWER BACK, STRENGTHENING THE CORE, AND INVERTING THE LEGS)

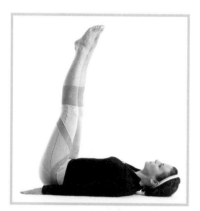

Lie on your back with your head and shoulders comfortably resting upon the floor. Arms relax down by your sides. Extend both legs up, forming an "L" with your body.

Exhale and lift the hips up overhead. Then inhale and *un*hinge at the hip, bringing the legs up toward the ceiling. Inhale, then exhale and return to the starting position. Repeat 5 (10, 15, 20) times total.

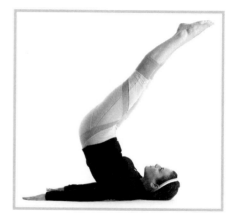

Scissors

(THIS PILATES EXERCISE IS AN INVERSION THAT REJUVENATES TIRED FEET, LEGS, AND HIPS;
IT'S ALSO GREAT FOR TONING THE THIGH MUSCLES)

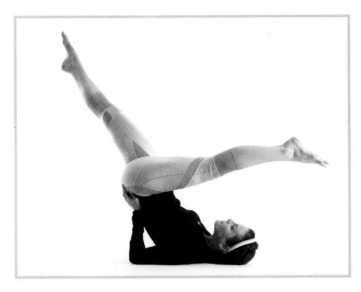

This exercise is performed in a shoulder stand position. To do this, lie on your back, with your head and shoulders resting comfortably on the floor, legs straight up toward the ceiling, and arms down by your sides. Exhale and lift your hips up and overhead. Press the palms of your hands into your lower back for support as you hike your legs up into what is known as a "shoulder stand."

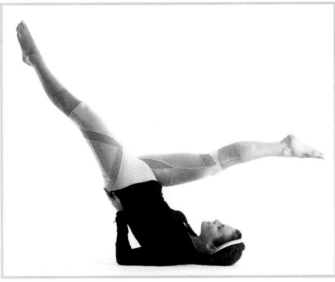

Point your toes and keep both legs straight as you scissor the right leg forward and the left leg back. Pause for a moment in a split-like stance, and then switch legs, bringing the left leg forward and the right leg back. Alternate at a steady pace for a total of 10 (20, 30, 40) repetitions. Then gracefully return the lower back to the floor and relax.

Neck Pull

*(THIS EXERCISE STRETCHES THE BACK,
FLATTENS THE BELLY, AND PROVIDES
A STRESS-RELIEVING OPPORTUNITY FOR THE NECK)*

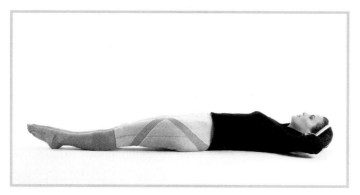

Lie on your back with your legs outstretched before you and both hands behind your head.

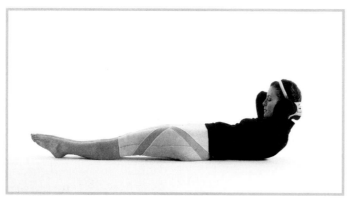

Exhale, curl the chin in toward the chest.

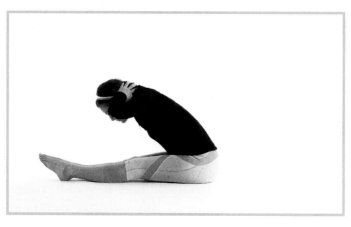

Continue to roll up into a seated position until you are curled all the way over. Inhale and pause momentarily, then exhale and smoothly roll down to the starting position. The legs remain grounded the entire time. Repeat 5 (10, 15, 20) times total.

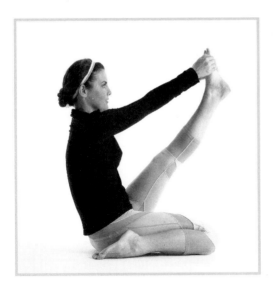

Heron Pose
(Krounchasana)

(THIS POSE BRINGS ENERGY INTO YOUR KNEE JOINTS AND PROVIDES A GOOD HAMSTRING STRETCH)

Sit upright with one knee bent behind you—the ankle is adjacent to your hip. Grab hold of the other leg, extend it, and pull it in toward your body. Hold here for 30 (60, 90, 120) seconds, then switch leg positions and repeat on the other side.

What's Ahead of Capricorn: A Star-Driven Five-Year Plan

2007   Feel the earth rumbling under your feet and something is telling you to prepare for big changes. You don't need to do anything yet, but you might want to rest, stay fit, and enjoy the status quo while you have it.
Key Workout: Cardio conditioning.

2008   Planetary energy hits your sign with full impact. You're ready for an amazing year. If you're prepared (healthy, positive, hopeful) you can have anything you want. Work, love, friendships—you're the one who can have it all.
Key Workout: Tennis.

2009   You're ready to reap the benefits from last year's powerful push. Money and work matters open up and your ability to invest is promising. Just don't spend more than you can afford.
Key Workout: Treadmill while watching CNN.

2010   Your career is your focus this year. You want to work hard and climb to another peak. You're fully prepared to make that trek but you'll need to pay attention to your social skills too. Goats aren't always interesting companions.

Key Workout: Walking with friends.

2011   Career rewards finally seem within your reach and you might consider relaxing at some point. Home is where the heart is; don't you want to spend more time there now? Your life is successful when you're happy, not tired.

Key Workout: Early morning runs.

Signs of Life

Capricorns work hard on all aspects of life. You're not all work and no play, though. Read up on the signs that rule different sectors of your chart and get to know yourself on other levels.

Love life—Cancer

Career—Libra

Flirtation—Taurus

Health—Gemini

aquarius-action

THE WATER BEARER January 20—February 18

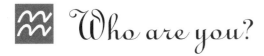 *Who are you?*

In One Word: VISIONARY

Symbol(s): Aquarius is a complex sign. Being The Water Bearer, many people assume that Aquarius is a water sign but actually it is an air sign. The Water Bearer stands as a vast figure in the universe, pouring water from a large urn into our world. We are fed ideas, innovation, invention, and radical shifts in reality from this ethereal water.

Color: Electric blue

Element: AIR. As the third and last air sign, you are the one who provides ideals and concepts. With pieces of information from Gemini, and balance and sense provided by Libra, Aquarius moves into brand new ideas and thoughts with a mind toward improving and progressing society. New fashion trends are started by Aquarians who abandon them once they catch on. Aquarians are government leaders (Ronald Reagan) and talk show hosts (Ellen DeGeneres, Oprah Winfrey). You'll also find that many teachers are Aquarians. The Water Bearer nourishes the mind.

Energy: FIXED. Aquarius is the last fixed sign of the zodiac and we believe you are the most fixed of them all. Of the four, Taurus has a reputation of being stubborn.

zodiaction

Leo has a reputation of being arrogant. Scorpio is unwilling and secretive. But Aquarius is boldly unmoving, sometimes even when it's obvious that you need to take that next step! Aquarians can be misunderstood in this way—you're the first to come up with radical new ideas but you can be the last to conform to the simplest task. Being fixed and unpredictable is an interesting combination.

Psychic Domain: You're one of the more psychic signs of the zodiac, ruled by the planet Uranus, which was discovered around the time of the American and French revolutions. You are an open socket for psychic impulses, which explains why you are so inventive and unpredictable. No one can tell you what to do. Even as a child, you were not interested in conforming to rules or standards. As an adult, you might have learned to look as if you belong in a crowd but inwardly you detest them. Although Aquarius rules groups and friendships, you are actually more comfortable in smaller clusters. You lead—you're a natural teacher, an inspiring speaker, a reluctant icon—but you're not looking for admiration. You're looking to make a difference.

Physical Domain: Aquarius rules the lower legs and ankles and is especially prone to sprains. Shin splints may also be a problem. Since Aquarius is ruled by the planet Uranus, you're sensitive to aura, atmosphere, and vibrations. You need to pay attention to your intuitive faculties as well as your physical body. Circulation can also be affected.

What to Avoid in the Aquarius Workout: The latest fad or a drill sergeant.

Ideal Workout: Full body stretching and cardio that helps you feel grounded and alive.

Essential Workout Gear: High quality, shock-absorbing shoes, and breathable, seamless socks.

Ultimate Trouble Spot: Ankles.

Workout Buddy Warning: Working out with someone isn't your first choice unless it is a trainer or a trusted old friend who can read you like Braille. You're just not consistently chatty. You keep yourself company by communing with your inner thoughts. Once in a while you'll enjoy a new person, perhaps on a walk or next to you on the recumbent bike. You're pretty good with strangers. Just be honest and upfront when you want to go it alone.

If You Have a Personal Trainer:

1. You're best with someone cute, quirky, and confident.

2. Atmosphere is everything—you *must* sense a good vibe.

3. You would do well with a trainer who has some interest in astrology or spiritual mind–body matters. Buzzwords include chakra, aura, and karma.

Strategic Choices for Aquarius

The Aquarian Diet: There is no reason to believe that you suddenly become a conformist when it comes to food. Aquarians have specific preferences, none of them predictable, all of them finicky. If you have a hankering for the perfect pastry, it must be from the French bakery of your choice, no matter how inconvenient it might be. If you're in the mood for a Philly cheesesteak, you would consider hopping a train to get it. You have your favorite things, and the rest is just fuel. Aquarians aren't usually overeaters. You're more selective and you don't like to overindulge. However, if you're feeling stifled, bored, or unable to find an audience to appreciate your ideas, you could end up "holding" energy in. Your sign rules auras, the energetic space around the body. Auras shift and change with every breath. You can expand your aura when you need to create more space between you and the world—or you can expand your waistline—sometimes both. If you find that you're prone to weight gain you need to look carefully at your emotional state. Are you fulfilled in your work and love life? Are you living in a way that allows you to be the truly unique individual that you are?

Aquarians need a voice. If you're not being heard, you could gain weight from frustration through overeating, drinking too much alcohol, or not sleeping well (or any combination of the three). Alcohol can take the edge off feeling misunderstood, but it's a dangerous and temporary fix. If you're not sleeping well, you'll need more fuel to get you through your day. It's a vicious cycle. If you're an overweight Aquarian, you need to change something in your life before you start a diet or you'll just gain the weight back.

zodiaction

1. **The season's freshest fruit.** Sure, fruit that is in season tends to taste better, but the Aquarian reason for selecting seasonal fruit is variety, so you won't get bored. Choose from berries and melon in spring, peaches and plums in summer, apples in autumn, and citrus over the winter.

2. **Dill pickles.** Salty, cold foods are very appealing to you. While anchovies and cheese are high fat options best indulged in moderation, pickles are pretty harmless and can safely satisfy this craving. (Olives are another option. They are high in fat, but it's the healthy, unsaturated kind.)

3. **Natural high mineral content water.** "Natural" mineral water is a legal definition meaning it comes from an identified and protected source, as opposed to "fortified." The Aquarian's ideal water should be rich in magnesium and calcium and have low sodium content. This type of water, which is thought to help cleanse one's aura, can be found in most markets—just read the label. It's not a bad idea to have your water tested at home to learn your current mineral content. Also, well water has a great track record for being high in minerals.

Diet Vice: Impulse buys at gourmet-to-go delis.
Signature Spa Treatment: Swedish massage.
Complementary Therapy: Aura cleansing and Reiki.
Mindfulness Mantra: If I stay grounded the world will be a better place.

Aquarius is the do-gooder humanitarian, we-are-the-world sign of the zodiac. You have scores of ideas on how to improve things, from fashion to schooling to government. The world according to Aquarian ideals would be a fabulous place to live. Unfortunately, your ideas aren't always practical (because you're five steps ahead of everyone else when you explain them), and you don't always take time to see them through.

You are inventive and even eccentric but you don't really notice how different you are. You are a staunch friend, natural peacekeeper, and a broad-thinking influencer. No one can tell you what to do and you hardly ever take any advice—sometimes to your own detriment. The world benefits from your Aquarian vision when you stay grounded enough to communicate what you see.

Aquarius in a Nutshell

MIND: Your large-scale, panoramic mind can take in a bird's eye view of any situation and you'll have more than one way to improve it. You're a teacher, philosopher, and champion of the human race. Let what's on your mind be known to the rest of us and you'll be doing some great work.

BODY: You do inhabit a body although you're not that interested in its details. Because you're more intellectual than physical, learning more about health and fitness would be a good thing. While you're naturally intuitive about many people and situations, you're not always in tune with your body. Let physical health be a new hobby and you'll stay fit and alert so that the world can benefit from your awesome mind—and everything else you have to offer.

SPIRIT: You see what can be and you lead us to it.

Share your visions, hopes, and wishes and the world will support them. Stay connected to the world around you so that your vision can be understood.

An Aquarian Workout Story

Jody was a soccer star in college for a top-ranked, Division I team and, like a lot of athletes, she immediately gained weight when it came time to hang up her jersey. In her five years since college, Jody has put on twenty-five pounds—which is a lot for a 5'3"-tall girl, who never had to worry about her weight.

The reason for Jody's weight gain *seems* obvious: her grueling, three-hour stints abruptly ended. After all, athletes get super-fit in the first place because they are forced to work out, right? They've got trainers and coaches making them move every day. The sudden lack of workout guidance is part of why Jody struggled with her weight post-college, but there is another reason too—an Aquarian reason.

Long before college, Jody's entire life was crammed with soccer. When she was eleven years old, she recalls setting the alarm clock for her four AM wake-up call and practice before school. She played year-round in multiple leagues. When she received a full collegiate scholarship, she celebrated for a moment, and then continued to train even harder. It's been a long road for Jody. When her four-year ride was up, it wasn't just the end of college; it was the end of a prison sentence. For the first time in her adult life, Jody was free.

Aquarians are freedom-loving, and for the majority of Jody's life, her freedom was compromised by a commitment to soccer. When Jody thought long and hard about her weight gain, she realized that it was actually an act of rebellion against the strict schedule she'd kept for most of her life.

So how should Jody go about getting in shape again? First, she must mentally, spiritually, and emotionally make peace with the past. Acknowledging the deeper reasons for her post-college weight woes is a big first step. Second, she needs to formulate a flexible exercise routine. (We suggest all Aquarians write their fitness plan in pencil, allowing for alterations along the way.)

THE AQUARIAN "NO PRESSURE" WORKOUT

Aquarians are notoriously bad followers. That's because you love your freedom and hate being told what to do. You can't possibly follow a fitness program if you feel hemmed in by rules. So the Aquarian workout is all about choice, options, and flexibility.

In essence, the Aquarius *No Pressure Workout* is a customized *non-plan.* Within its subtle structure resides room for impulses, personal preferences, and daydreaming. Each section is an energy-enhancing blitz in and of itself, so your workout can be one step, two steps, or all three. "Just do something every day" is the motto we'd like to set for you, Aquarius. Your workouts need not be long, intense, or memorable. They simply have to *be.* For you, moving clears away the clutter in your head, connects you to the here-and-now, and focuses your attention. Three good reasons to keep on reading!

Step 1 is called *Elemental Cardio,* where fifteen minutes of just about anything that gets your heart rate up is welcome. You have a huge selection to choose from within the four elements–*fire, earth, water,* and *air.* Step 2 is called *Circle Strength,* where big circular movements come into play. Here, we multitask as we tone, hitting all of the major muscles of the body in just five exercises, which can be performed in any order, and with either hand weights, wrist weights, or a medicine ball. Step 3 is *Quirky Stretch.* You're drawn to the unconventional, so these five unorthodox stretches will suit you well.

THREE WORKOUT GOALS FOR AQUARIUS

1. Energize the whole being, body, mind, and spirit.

2. Gain a sense of freedom by big ranges of motion, limited equipment, and a flexible plan.

3. Reduce/manage stress with focused stretching technique.

WORKOUT PRESCRIPTION

Aquarians need to feel in control. You're not about power-mongering—you're about individuality. You can't be told what to do or even how to do it. You need to fulfill your whims and needs and no one knows what they are better than you.

We'll take a cue from Oprah, an Aquarian born on the 29th of January. She fluctuated from a habitual exerciser to habitual non-exerciser, marathoner to couch potato. (Aquarius is a fixed sign, so ruts are very possible.) She's learned the hard way that one needs to keep at it, day by day. We've given you many options in *Zodiaction*. You can go full throttle for a hardcore workout, mix and match for a good overall energizer, or opt for the just-get-by minimum for a quick pick-me-up. As long as you do something, you'll be just fine.

BEST TIME TO WORK OUT: Whenever the mood strikes (as long as the mood hits no less than three times a week!).

STEP 1: Elemental Cardio. Okay, Water Bearer, let's get to it. The four elements of the zodiac make their way into your cardiovascular plan of action. First up is your element, *Air*. Some great examples of *Air* cardio include trampoline rebounding, running, and jumping rope. The focus here is on lightness, breath, and up-energy. Think of a helium balloon floating upward in the sky.

Next, *Water* cardio includes swimming, aqua-robics, and canoeing. Notice the fluidity of movement and the gentle muscular resistance that water brings. Water has a calming effect on the psyche too, so these types of cardio activities are perfect if your nervous system needs a little soothing!

Earth cardio includes activities like hiking, walking, and power yoga. It's all about connecting to the ground, so truly notice how your foot rolls from toe to heel while hiking, or how the palms of your hands are rooted to the floor while performing Downward-Facing Dog.

zodiaction

The fourth element, *Fire*, includes seriously sweaty, heat-provoking activities like sprinting, cycling, and Tae-Bo. Witness how the heat rises in your body and your blood seemingly pulses through your veins. The two absolutes for Step 1 are:

1. Make it fifteen minutes in duration. That's what it takes to make an impact.

2. Periodically, connect to the dominant element during the activity, by mentally reminding yourself it's there. It'll add a layer of depth to your workout—keeping it interesting for Aquarians.

STEP 2: Circle Strength. It's time to work on strengthening your body, but don't worry, there are no confining Nautilus machines involved! You'll master five big-range-of-motion exercises that provide freedom of movement and condition multiple muscle groups at once. This routine can be performed with hand weights, wrist weights, or a medicine ball, and in any order.

Torso Circle

(STRENGTHENS THE MUSCLES OF THE LEGS, CORE, AND ARMS)

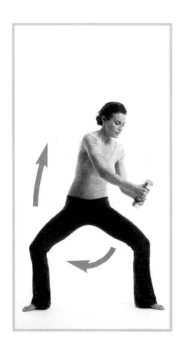 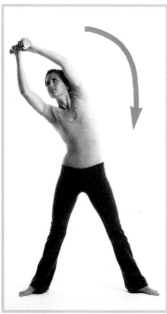

Stand with your feet approximately four feet apart, toes slightly turned out, knees bent. Grasp the weights with both hands and engage your core muscles.

Exhale and move your arms in a circle as if tracing a big clock. Begin at the bottom, circle around up to the top, and then around to the starting position. Repeat ten times clockwise, then ten additional times counterclockwise.

Overhead Lasso

(STRENGTHENS THE MUSCLES OF THE UPPER BODY)

Stand with your feet approximately four feet apart, toes slightly turned out. Extend out both arms, like airplane wings. Hold a weight in each hand.

Circle the right arm up and around, making a big "halo" overhead. You should feel a subtle backbend and stretch to the chest, as well as toning in the arms and torso. Repeat ten times, and then repeat ten additional times with the left hand.

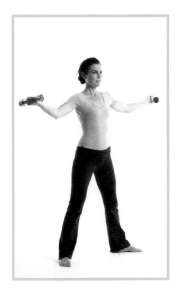 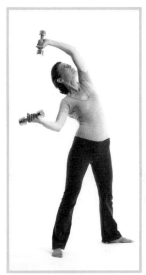

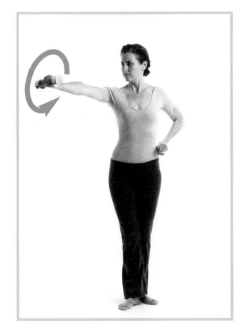

Diagonal Arm Circle

(STRENGTHENS THE ARM MUSCLES)

Stand tall with feet together. Extend your right arm out to a diagonal angle, at shoulder level. Hold one weight in your right hand, as you maintain a firm wrist and a slight micro-bend in your right elbow. Simply rotate the arm in a circle the size of a dinner plate. Rotate ten times in each direction (clockwise and counterclockwise), then repeat the series with the left arm at a diagonal.

Standing Leg Circle

(STRENGTHENS THE BUTT AND THIGH MUSCLES)

Stand tall with hands resting upon hips. Extend your right leg out directly to the side, point the toes, and maintain a straight leg, if possible. All of your weight is distributed on your left leg. Simply rotate the leg in a circle as if tracing a Frisbee. Rotate ten times in each direction (clockwise and counterclockwise), then switch sides and perform the exercise again on the other side.

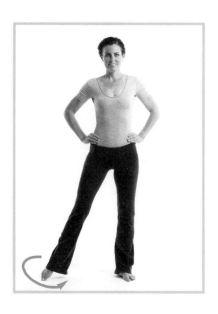

Wrap Twist

(STRENGTHENS, STRETCHES, AND RELEASES TENSION IN THE MUSCLES OF THE CORE)

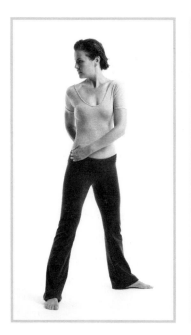
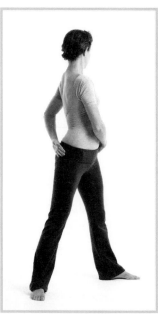

Stand with your feet approximately four feet apart. Toes are slightly turned out and the legs are as straight and active as possible. Keep your spine straight.

Exhale and twist the torso to the left, reaching the right arm across to the left hip bone. Then exhale and twist the torso to the right, reaching the left arm across to the right hip bone. Alternate side to side for a total of twenty repetitions.

STEP 3: Quirky Stretch. These stretches may appear awkward, but they definitely get the job done. They present an excellent balance challenge, core challenge, and muscular stretch in each and every one. These six stretches can be performed in any order.

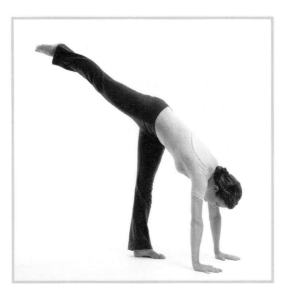

Forward Bend Scissor

(TARGETS THE HAMSTRINGS)

Stand with feet together and bend forward. Place your hands on the floor in front of you, but try to rely on these as little as possible—this will make you balance, use your core, and tune in. At this point, kick the right leg up as high as it can go. Hold here for 30–60 seconds, and then perform the identical stretch on the other side.

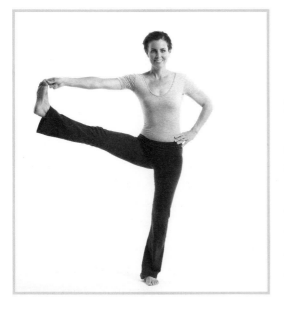

Standing Side Straddle

(TARGETS THE INNER THIGH)

Stand tall with both feet together. Reach down with your right hand and grab hold of the right foot. Using balance and core strength, lift the leg up and over to the right. Try to make the leg as straight as possible and keep the spine as erect as possible. Hold here for 30–60 seconds, and then perform the identical stretch on the other side.

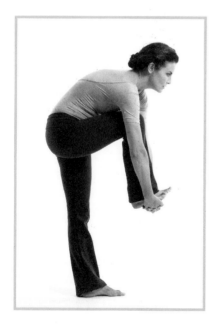

90-Degree Knee Stretch

(TARGETS THE MUSCLES OF THE LOWER BACK)

Engage your core muscles by pulling the navel toward your spine, balance on your left foot, and grab the right foot with both hands. Bring the right thigh upward and obtain a 90-degree angle at the right knee. The standing leg is fully extended. Hold here for 30–60 seconds, and then perform the identical stretch on the other side.

Cross-Legged Reverse Plank

(TARGETS THE CHEST AND THIGHS)

Sit cross-legged with a tall spine. Place the palms of your hands directly underneath your shoulders, fingers pointing away from you. Gracefully lift your hips up off the ground, keeping the spine straight. (Be sure not to throw your head back.) Hold here for 30–60 seconds and then gracefully release.

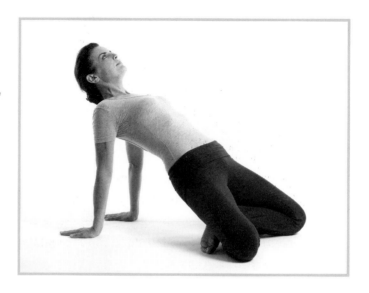

Dancer's Drama Stretch

(TARGETS THE WHOLE SIDE BODY)

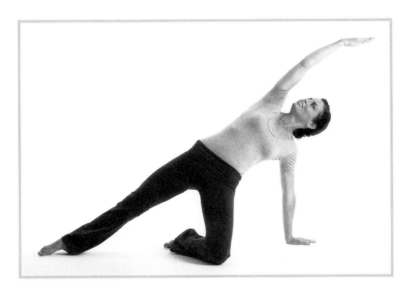

Sit with your right leg extended out and left leg bent in, the sole of the left foot pressing lightly against the right inner thigh. You'll be supported by your left arm, so place it directly underneath the left shoulder for proper alignment. Now simply lift the hips up off the floor while reaching the right arm up and overhead. Hold for 30–60 seconds, release, and repeat the exercise with the left leg extended.

What's Ahead of Aquarius: A Star-Driven Five-Year Plan

2007   It's all about your self-vision. What do you see in your future? You're going to make great headway this year if you put your mind to it, or rather, put your feet to it. You have the ideas, now make them real.
Key Workout: African dance is very grounding.

2008   Things are going on behind the scenes and you are positively psychic on a daily basis. You're working on big changes and the universe is cooperating. It's not the best year to dig in your heels so rethink all habits and every time you say "no," try to think through the possibility of "yes."
Key Workout: Yoga.

2009   Now that cosmic energy is fully on your side, you must make the most of it. No more "what if" or "if only." You're ready to achieve some big goals and if you don't totally go for it, you have no one to blame. Feel the pressure? Good.

Key Workout: Kickboxing.

2010   Hopefully you're in a position to capitalize on the progress you made last year. You're ready for more of everything—money, friends, love, or property. You name it, you can build toward your dreams. Opt for staying close to home and working on your life rather than flying off on trips or going off to daydreams.

Key Workout: Power walking.

2011   The planets might challenge you in communications this year, so it's going to be important to be clear with your friends and family. It's a great idea to clear your head before you express any major new idea or opinion, so keep your workout schedule consistent. You want to stay grounded and make sense.

Key Workout: At-home exercise DVDs.

Signs of Life

Aquarians are obstinate individualists by nature, but your chart doesn't stop there. Your life has paradoxical and complementary signs that give you more dimension and sometimes even more consistency (and that's not a bad thing). Read the following signs to get more insight into your unique cosmic structure.

Love life—Leo

Career—Taurus

Flirtation—Gemini

Health—Cancer

pisces-action

THE FISH February 19–March 20

 Who are you?

In One Word: IDEALISTIC

Symbol(s): Pisces is an extremely spiritual and creative sign. The fish has been a symbol of eternal spirit long before Christianity adopted it as a representation of Jesus Christ. The astral symbol of Pisces is actually two fish swimming in opposite directions. Like fellow water sign Cancer, the fish incorporates the duality of existence, the yin and the yang, light and dark, conscious and unconscious.

Color: Pale violet or sea green (depending on your mood)

Element: WATER. You are the third and final water sign and the last sign of the zodiac. You are the epitome of "still waters run deep," although you do your best to hide your depths. As a fish, you have no way to protect yourself from the world's vibes. When things are good, you swim in bliss. You know the world can be a terrifying place but you lack the defense mechanisms that can protect your fellow water signs. Cancer can retreat into its shell and The Scorpion's sting is a strong deterrent to ocean predators. You have neither and, as a result of being vulnerable, you tend to anesthetize yourself instead of learning to fight back. That's the price you pay for being the deepest, most psychic sign.

Energy: MUTABLE. Pisces shifts and surfs, twists and turns with ease. You prefer to dream than to listen to hard facts. You create and imagine in your heart when others build or problem-solve with their hands. When you do set your mind to something you can get almost anything done—as long your efforts promise a measure of pleasure or reward. You can charm the shell off a lobster and the teeth out of a shark. You just don't apply yourself that often.

Psychic Domain: Think dolphins: the sea mammals that are intelligent, friendly, playful, and, as many believe, psychic. Of course, the world is a tough place for a friendly sea creature. Your deep-sea psyche and penetrating intuition can be overwhelmed by simple everyday life. You always need private time, sleep, and escapism if you're going to function well. You can't be in a screamingly loud environment for too long but you do love to venture out for inspiration. The arts, poetry, and music in all forms are ruled by Pisces. You create, withdraw, and regenerate.

Physical Domain: Pisces rules the feet, liver, and lymphatic system. Your feet are so important because they carry you where you want to go, keep you grounded, and take on your physical weight. Since Pisceans love a bit of escapism, watch out for the alcohol. Your liver is not able to process a lot of it.

What to Avoid in the Pisces Workout: Aggressive crowds and crashing music.

Ideal Workout: Swimming.

Essential Workout Gear: A flattering and functional bathing suit. You want to look good but the priority should be a suit that supports your water work over sunbathing.

Ultimate Trouble Spot: Arches and soles of feet.

Workout Buddy Warning: A workout buddy is only good for keeping you focused on your fitness program or talking to you about one of your pet projects. If you have a life that is crowded with communications and business, work out alone or with someone who doesn't talk too much. Your workout can become your very necessary "alone time."

If You Have a Personal Trainer:

1. Choose a woman. You need that gentle-but-firm nurturing quality that will most likely be found in a female.

2. When it comes to booking sessions, don't be too aggressive. Once a week is just enough to keep a Pisces on track. Play it by ear week to week. A long-term, hard commitment may feel overwhelming. (As a mutable sign, you just can't predict where you'll be next Tuesday, anyway.)

3. Make sure your trainer provides you with a full-body program.

Strategic Choices for Pisces

The Piscean Diet: The first person to order another bottle of wine might be the Sagittarian but the one who finishes the last glass is the Pisces. You won't be the one who orders the chocolate mousse either, but your spoon will visit the plate more than once. You are someone who cannot say no to pleasure. Whatever your preferences are—cheese, bread, chocolate, beer, pasta, nachos, or all of the above—you enjoy your food. It is a gift to enjoy the small pleasures of a great taste, but it is a problem when you can't stop yourself. Pisces isn't the most overindulgent, it's just the most innocent. You don't stop to think about what you're doing when you're having a good time.

If you are emotionally even and clear, you won't have any diet worries. The danger occurs when you are feeling low, vulnerable, angry, anxious, or sad. You might eat, drink, or smoke to escape or to feed your happiness.

First, because Pisces rules the feet and the liver, you need to take care of your diet. Excess weight equals excess strain on your feet, which can lead to swelling and fatigue. Over time you may develop more serious orthopedic problems, causing pain when you do try to exercise. Swimming is a great way to relieve pressure on your feet as well as a great way to stay slim.

Second, your ultra-sensitive liver finds it difficult to process foods rich in fat, fried foods, and animal-based proteins like eggs, dairy, and meat. Alcohol and coffee also put a strain on your liver's functions. Your friends and colleagues might be able to drink coffee all day, and then sip wine all evening without much consequence, but you cannot. Your energy level and waistline will pay a big price, so don't follow their lead. You don't have to be a saint. You just need to set limits and find ways to continually cleanse your insides.

zodiaction

THE TOP THREE ITEMS TO SHOP FOR:

1. Lemon. Lemons have an astringent effect on the liver and colon. Squeeze one-quarter of a fresh lemon in a cup of hot water for a great wake-up elixir (perhaps as a replacement for your morning coffee). You know those people who always have a beautiful bowl of lemons displayed in their kitchens? Be one of those people. If lemons are around, you'll use 'em!

2. Pomegranate juice. The bottle of juice at your fancy grocer may seem expensive, but we think it's worth the extra bucks. Pomegranate, the fruit and its juice, is known as a "super food" for a very good reason: there are huge amounts of health-creating antioxidants in the pomegranate. In the U.S., pomegranates are a fall fruit, so they tend to be hard to come by in the other seasons. This is why we advocate the juice, which is easy to find all year long. And hey, it still costs less than a Starbucks venti cappuccino, so, when you need energy or feel a cold coming on, splurge on brands like POM Wonderful.

3. The five "C's": carrots, cauliflower, celery, chives, and cucumber. These foods help keep the liver clean, which, in turn, helps maintain proper fat metabolism.

Diet Vice: Potato chips.
Signature Spa Treatment: Reflexology.
Complementary Therapy: Liver detoxification programs.
Mindfulness Mantra: If I set boundaries my world will be safe and happy.

Pisces is a sign that holds infinite love and forgiveness but lacks edge and limits. As creative and sensitive as you are, you can be equally numb and indifferent. That's what happens when you can't take it anymore.

The world benefits from your Piscean vision when you stay grounded enough to communicate what you see and you don't lose yourself in worrying about all the woes you perceive.

Pisces in a Nutshell

MIND: You like to use your third eye—the mind's psychic center where your inner vision lives—rather than your rational brain centers. Pisces isn't about left-brain or right-brain thinking; you're more like full-brain dreaming.

BODY: Most of the time you're at home in your body, a place that anchors you in this world and provides a bit of pleasure if not safety. You're a fluid being, soft and gentle on the outside, much more complex on the inside. You are highly intuitive about your health and you know when you're ignoring signs that you're unwell. You will learn to take care of your body one way or another. Make it the easy way and stay healthy.

SPIRIT: When you share your dreams you make the world a better place.

Allow yourself to act on your desires and you will fill your heart with joy. The world is a place where love connects and heals all fear.

A Piscean Workout Story

Have you ever wondered how some people love a certain exercise craze, while others abhor it? Gia, a Pisces born February 28, 1980, sure did when she stumbled into a raucous kickboxing class one rainy Tuesday. She couldn't take her normal stroll through Central Park, so going to the gym was the only available option.

Right from the start of class, the movements were jarring. The instructor was shouting. The music was blaring. From Gia's Piscean point of view, everything about the class was disturbing. She didn't realize Hell was located so close to her New York City apartment.

When Gia returned home from her first and last kickboxing class, she was eager to soak in the tub and forget about her experience, but two questions baffled her: Who was taking that class? And who was enjoying it? She just didn't understand how punching and kicking had become a popular form of fitness. Well, to answer both her questions: Millions of people. People from all walks of life adore kickboxing. Male or female, old or young, fit or unfit. (We think plenty of Aries and Scorpios too!)

The bottom line is this: Gia is a genuine Pisces. She needs soothing, nonviolent fitness options that create a serene buzz inside and out. She should stick with those walks in Central Park and eschew anything with a *jab, punch,* or *hook* in its vocabulary.

THE PISCES "DREAMY" WORKOUT

Pisceans will take little notice of intense exercise when it involves something pleasurable or diverting. Music, beautiful countryside, the ability to be lost in your head—these all make working out a lot easier. In fact, you wouldn't call it working out—more like chilling out with a good heart rate. You will stay fit as long as you're not being subjected to boredom or pain. Pisces proves that *no pain, no gain* is a myth when the workout environment is appealing.

Pisceans love to visit la-la land, and this three-step workout can take you there. Step 1, *Single-Nostril Breathing,* is perfect for those days where your energy reserve is low and your stress levels are high. Step 2, *Swimming,* will get you into the water for your cardio. It's easy on your feet and feels like home. Step 3 is *Gentle Seated Yoga,* where working out isn't war, it's pure peace.

The Pisces *Dreamy Workout* must be performed in order, but only two out of the three need to be performed. One section can always be tossed to the side and saved for another day. So on Monday, do *Single-Nostril Breathing* and *Swimming.* Tuesday will find you back in the pool for *Swimming,* and then *Gentle Seated Yoga.* Wednesday, *Single-Nostril Breathing,* followed by gentle yoga.

THREE WORKOUT GOALS FOR PISCES

1. Stretch the body and divert the mind.

2. Use cardio as an excuse to listen to music or drift off into dreamland.

3. Concentrate on tone, not strength.

WORKOUT PRESCRIPTION

Pisceans are not big thrill-seekers or weekend warriors. You can stick with a routine as long as it doesn't seem like a commitment to suffer. Swimming lulls you into a peaceful place, a treadmill with a nice view zens you into a dream zone, and a walk in the countryside wouldn't feel like fitness at all. You need to find a way to enjoy what you're doing so that it doesn't feel like work. Forget barking instructors or boot-camp tactics.

BEST TIME TO WORK OUT: Midday so you can fit in a little daydreaming during work hours.

STEP 1: Single-Nostril Breathing. Breathing is the foundation for life and the foundation for all exercise. It clears the stale air from the lungs and saturates the cells with oxygen. It helps remove impurities from the blood, and tones up the circulatory and respiratory systems, as well as the abdominal muscles. For Pisces, breathing is the supreme soother, in body, mind, and spirit. Find a quiet place, kick off your shoes, and give yourself ten minutes to sit still and focus on your breath.

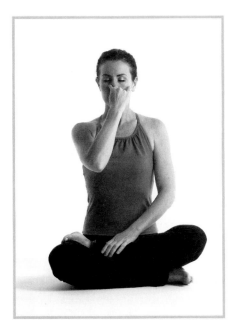

Sit comfortably in a seated cross-legged position. Your spine and neck should be straight with your ears directly over your shoulders. (The alignment of your spine is crucial. If you find it difficult to maintain, feel free to sit up against a wall for support.) Softly close your eyes and bring the right hand up to the nose. Use the fingers of your right hand to close off each nostril, alternately. Hold them in a position called "Vishnu Mudra." To establish "Vishnu Mudra," extend the thumb and little finger of your right hand and fold down your other three fingers into your palm. Rest the left hand on your left leg. Close the right nostril with the thumb, and breathe through the left nostril. Inhale through the left nostril to a slow count of three. Exhale to a count of six. Repeat ten times. Then breathe through the right nostril. Close the left nostril with the pinky finger, and inhale through the right nostril to a slow count of three. Exhale to a count of six. Repeat ten times total then slowly open your eyes.

STEP 2: Swimming. You feel at home in and around water, so why not make it a cardio staple? Find a local pool and research its lap-swim hours. *Allocate two or three days per week to a one mile, cardiovascular swim.* (Most high school and college pools have lap lengths of twenty-five yards per lap. One mile will be seventy-one laps, there and back.) A key component to making your swim a success is having an unrushed, easy mind-set before you dive in. Take a break when you need to. Switch up your stroke from freestyle to butterfly whenever you feel the need. Don't use a stopwatch, it'll only stress you out; you're not swimming for time anyway, you're swimming for length. One cute, kind mile.

STEP 3: Gentle Seated Yoga. If there was ever an activity that un-frazzled the frazzled, it's gentle yoga. The following seven poses are seated (easy on your feet, Pisces) and meant to be non-strenuous (easy on your nerves). If a pose feels too tough, skip it, and move on to the next. Now just kick off your shoes, grab a mat, play some mellow tunes, and do yoga.

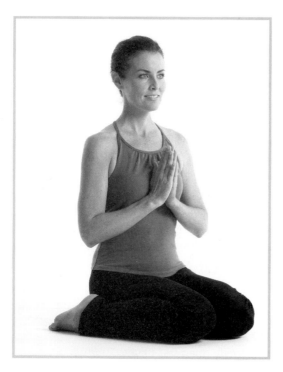

Hero's Pose
(Virasana)

(HERO'S POSE BRINGS RELIEF TO TIRED LEGS)

Kneel on your mat with both knees together. Keeping your back tall and straight, push your shins out, and sit down between the ankles. Use your hands for support if necessary. Hold for one minute and then gracefully release.

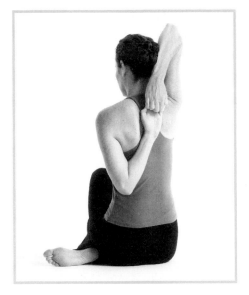

Cow-Faced Pose (Gomukhasana)

(THIS POSE STRETCHES THE ANKLE AREA, HIP AREA, AND TRICEPS)

Sit on your mat and cross the left knee over the right. Try to stack the knees, one atop the other. Reach your right arm up and your left arm down and clasp the hands behind you, all the while keeping your spine straight and upright. Hold for sixty seconds and then repeat on the other side.

Plow Pose (Halasana)

(PLOW POSE REDUCES TENSION IN THE LOWER BACK)

Lie on your back with your head and shoulders comfortably resting on your mat, arms relaxed down at your sides. Slowly extend both legs up and overhead using a bit of core strength. You can bend the knees if you'd like. Once your toes make light contact with the floor, hold for one minute.

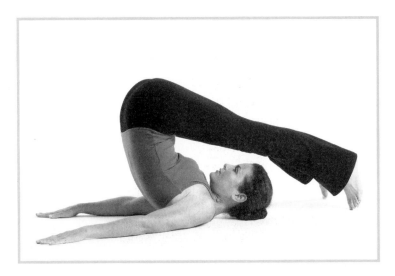

Seated Forward Bend (Paschimottanasana)

(SEATED FORWARD BEND IS AN AMAZING STRETCH FOR THE HAMSTRINGS AND LOWER BACK)

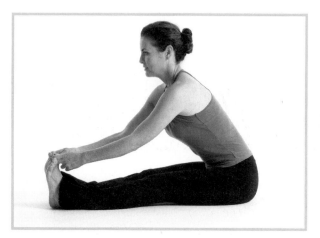

Sit on your mat with both legs extended out in front of you. Inhale and extend the body up, exhale and reach forward. Grab hold of your shins, ankles, or feet and gently pull your torso down. Hold for one minute.

Happy Baby Pose (Ananda Balasana)

(THIS POSE IS A PEACEFUL HIP OPENER)

Lie on your back with your head and shoulders comfortably resting on the mat. Bring your knees to your chest and grab hold of *the yogi toe lock*, where the index and middle fingers loop around the big toe of each foot. Your legs should form a 90-degree angle at the knees. Make sure your head and shoulders stay on the mat. Feet should be flexed, and your hips should be pressed down toward the mat. Hold for one minute.

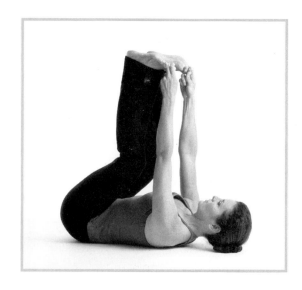

Fish Pose (Matsyasana)

(FISH POSE IS A SUBTLE INVERSION THAT SOOTHES THE NERVOUS SYSTEM BY BRINGING FRESH BLOOD TO THE BRAIN; IT ALSO OPENS THE HEART CHAKRA MAKING IT EASIER TO INHALE AND EXPAND THE LUNGS)

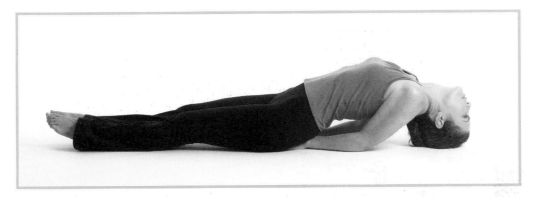

Lie on your back with your legs extended and your arms by your sides. Relax your head and shoulders completely, and keep your eyes open. Now gracefully crawl your hands (palms facing down) underneath your hips. As you walk your elbows in so they are in line with the wrists, your upper torso will lift up, allowing you to place the crown of your head on the floor. Hold for one minute.

Arrowhead

(THIS POSE IS A PEACEFUL HIP OPENER AND SIMPLE INNER THIGH STRETCH)

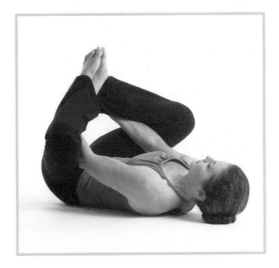

Lie on your back with your head resting comfortably on the ground. Grab your ankles by reaching in front of your knees, then match the soles of the feet together. Without lifting your head off the ground, pull your feet toward your chest. The elbows can help press the knees back. Hold for one minute.

Traditional Child's Pose (Balasana)

(CHILD'S POSE IS A GENTLE STRETCH FOR THE UPPER, MIDDLE, AND LOWER BACK)

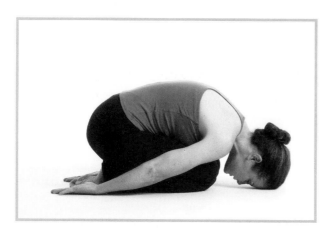

Kneel on your mat with ankles and knees touching. Sit on your heels and smoothly drape your torso forward, over your thighs. Your forehead should rest comfortably on the mat, while your arms remain down by your sides. Relax here for one minute, focusing on your calm inhalations and exhalations.

What's Ahead of Pisces: A Star-Driven Five-Year Plan

2007 Planetary energy in your career sector is keeping you on your toes. Swim through the obstacles by staying clear and focused. With Saturn meddling in your house of healthy snacks, you could binge. Back away from the chips and margaritas and hit the pool instead!
Key Workout: Lap swimming.

2008 Relationships are highlighted for the next two years and the energy to make the right love work cannot be denied. Thankfully star power shines in your dreams-come-true sector, so you'd better be in shape for your fairy-godmother's dress—they run small.
Key Workout: Ballet.

2009 The heavens conspire to make you very psychic this year. Since you're already amply gifted, in 2009 you're positively uncanny. Use your intuition to guide you through the tangle of relationships you're in and know that when the right change presents itself, you'll open the right door.
Key Workout: Flexibility training.

2010   Cosmic energy rolls into your sign this year. You can expand your power, your network, even your net worth—but that waistline can expand too with all the celebrating you could do. It's a joyful year. Make it a fit year too.
Key Workout: Water aerobics.

2011   Having money is a great thing. Spending it can be even more fun. But be careful not to get carried away. You don't need to carry on last year's exuberance to the point of testing your credit limit. Take risks with your heart, not your plastic.
Key Workout: At-home exercise DVDs.

Signs of Life

Pisceans are obstinate individualists by nature, but your chart doesn't stop there. Your life has paradoxical and complementary signs that give you more dimension and sometimes even more consistency (and that's not a bad thing). Read the chapters on the following signs to get more insight into your unique cosmic structure.

    Love life—Leo

    Career—Taurus

    Flirtation—Gemini

    Health—Cancer

Index

index

index

ABOUT THE AUTHORS

ELLEN BARRETT is the star of four bestselling exercise DVDs, an instructor on FIT TV, and owns the mind/body/fitness center The Studio by Ellen Barrett.

BARRIE DOLNICK is a nationally acclaimed astrologer and author.

Both authors live in New Haven, Connecticut.